Live a VIBRANT LIFE!®

Dawn King and Robert King

ICAN Press ✦ Vernon, B.C. Canada

The purpose of this book is to share our personal experiences with respect to enhancing health and the use of nutritional supplements. No part of this book is intended, nor should it be interpreted, as diagnostic or prescriptive. The body heals itself and its ability to do so is enhanced by nutritional supplements.

We believe in a wholistic approach to health. This book promotes the notion of being a self-responsible citizen living in a global community. *Live a Vibrant Life* is intended to educate, entertain, and empower.

ICAN Press
P.O. Box 1720
Vernon, B.C. Canada
V1T 8C3

First edition • Printed in Canada
ISBN: 0-9780710-0-X

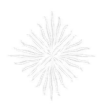

The information in this book takes you back to the basics of health, leading you through ways to build your health foundation by establishing your biological homeostasis (balance). Unfortunately, in the scientific and medical publishing world the concept of K.I.S.S. seems to have been totally forgotten, and information is often confusing and convoluted. This book presents logical, understandable steps to help you obtain your optimum spiritual and physical health.

–Dr. Kurt Grange, Ph.D., N.D., Nutritional Biophysiologist

Live a vibrant life! This says it all. Today many people are living a physical and spiritual nightmare—due to stress, environmental toxins, diets high in fat and sugar, smoking, soft drinks, abuse of pharmaceutical drugs, etc.—and are trapped there because of lack of knowledge. This book offers the keys to getting control of your physical and spiritual self. Through supplementation and detoxification, learn how to alkalize, cleanse, nourish, and balance your body. Follow this step-by-step approach to achieving wellness and you too will live a vibrant life!

–Dr. Jeff Bennert, Ph.D., CTN

Dedicated to the many inspiring and forward-thinking natural health pioneers, and all those who advocate living a vibrant, healthy life! To our teachers, students, and clients, as Dawn would say: "Shine on!"

Contents

Acknowledgments

It takes a team to undertake an adventure like this one! There are many players involved, some directly and some more indirectly. To all of them (and you know who you are) please accept our profound gratitude and appreciation. Our contributions would be diminished without yours. Together we are stronger and can offer more to a world in need of healing.

As we look back on the journey this book has provided, we can recount many different emotions—excitement, frustration, gratitude, awe, certainty, and uncertainty, to name a few. We have a deep respect and admiration for the amazing, important research done by so many others. The fellowship and mentorship offered by like-minded individuals along the way have proven invaluable to us and for that we are deeply thankful. We are inspired by some very special way showers who we think of as "angels on earth." Likewise we deeply appreciate the support offered by colleagues, friends, and most importantly, family. To all of you, please accept our deepest gratitude.

We want to acknowledge the contributions of the many pioneers and proponents of natural and wholistic health and all those who have held the vision of a healthier, safer, and peaceful planet. We also want to acknowledge those who motivate and encourage themselves and others (including us) to realize our physical, mental, emotional, and spiritual potential.

In addition we want to acknowledge the personal contributions and support of these exceptional people ... Sandy and Ray Duff, Kathi Dunn and Ron "Hobie" Hobart, Grammy and Grandpa Dave,

Kimberley Lloyd, Dr. Clinton Howard, Dan Poytner, Dr. Jeff Bennert, and Dr. Kurt Grange. We are so grateful to our interior designer and copy editor, Sara Patton, who provided a lot of expertise and tender love and care. We are sure you will feel her incredible talents and gifts on every page. Thanks to you all, for believing in our project and our life's work.

Preface

We are delighted to offer this book to you. While it focuses on Dawn's many years as a health practitioner, professional speaker, and seminar leader with countless clients, it actually represents more than forty years of our combined experience working, learning, and growing in the helping professions.

The main idea for this book was conceived while we were living in Shanghai, China. We wanted to accomplish several things with it. Our plan was to offer our clients a simple, easy-to-follow, up-to-date tool—a roadmap and a system for success. Our intention was to develop an easy way of looking at healthy living as well as the critical need for supplementation and positive lifestyle choices. Our goal was to offer clear explanations to the questions we are so often asked. It was our desire to make those explanations entertaining, empowering, educational, and easy to duplicate.

We decided to write the book from Dawn's perspective as if she were talking (Dawn loves to talk!) because our intention was to make the book more conversational and fun. The book has truly been a joint labor of love, with Robert doing the bulk of the writing and Dawn offering the creativity and most of the anecdotal insights and stories.

It is our goal that this book will help you improve your health, regardless of your current level of wellness and fitness. (By the way, our 10-year-old daughter has also completed a book which she wrote entirely on her own. It is a delightful book with brilliant illustrations and offers a kid's perspective on a happy and healthy life.)

We are creating a book series that will inspire the emotional, mental, and spiritual aspects of living a healthy, vibrant life. Find out more about these books at www.DawnandRobertKing.com. The door is always open to our hearts and our "home" page!

As you travel along the royal highway to health, may your days be filled with peace, passion, purpose, play—and awesome health!

Live a vibrant life!

Dawn and Robert King

Vernon, B.C. Canada

August 2006

Introduction

This is a book for those who want to improve their health on every level and experience and live a vibrant life. It is a practical book written for those who want to improve or regain their health first and discuss the philosophies of health later.

After 20 years of helping thousands of people overcome illness, chronic postural pain, and disease, the recipe remains the same. As long as we respect the extraordinary powers of our mind, body, emotions, spirit, and nutritional sciences we will be blessed with incredible returns. How might things be better if we lived a vibrant life in a body free of illness, disease, and pain? The power and ability of our body to remain healthy and to restore health are incredible!

It doesn't matter where we live on the planet today. Cardiovascular disease (CVD) is the #1 killer. Of all male deaths in Canada in 2002, 32% were due to heart disease (Heart and Stroke Foundation of Canada, Statistics Canada 2002). The cost of this is staggering. According to Health Canada's 1998 report, "Economic Burden of Illness in Canada," cardiovascular diseases cost the Canadian economy over $18 billion per year! In the U.S. the rates of CVD are higher and the costs are becoming prohibitive. Cancer and diabetes are right behind.

This is not nature's way. There are no germs creating arthritis, fibromyalgia, colitis, or ADHD. You don't "catch" CVD, cancer, diabetes, or high blood pressure. But there is untold, unnecessary suffering for individuals, families, and communities who suffer these life-altering diseases. It is mind-boggling and ironic for so many people to choose death by lifestyle.

The answers are right in front of our noses, eyes, ears, and mouths. What we eat, think, believe, feel, and do is under our direct control. We can change for the better. Yet millions upon millions of our fellow humans choose to live unhealthy lives on a daily basis. We want to be part of the solution!

When Dawn was asked about her personal health journey, she replied, "Over twenty years ago, when my family's health was in jeopardy, I read a life-changing book: Dr. Zehr's *Healthy Steps*. I studied that book carefully and took consistent actions. My old ways of thinking and behaving had only provided my family and me with low energy and poor health. I changed my thinking and my behaviors. Every part of my health and life changed and improved!"

In this book you will find critical steps for living a healthy, vibrant life. A healthy, vibrant life is *the real you*. You need only to open your mind to what is possible and then take action. We have worked with countless clients who have achieved the results they wanted and overcome their previous and perceived limitations. So will you.

We believe in self-responsibility in all aspects of life. The bottom line is each of us is responsible for our own health. We also believe in teamwork, so we support the idea of a team of health practitioners to help when needed and to support our health. Healthy living takes dedication. While it does not seem to be the common path today, we see more and more people choosing to take charge of their own health. These people are educating themselves about nutrition, supplementation, and lifestyle, and making positive, life-supportive choices and changes. We salute you.

While we were working through the drafts of this book we received feedback and suggestions from many people, for which we are very grateful. One of the ideas was to include a list of ailments and illnesses and Dawn's preferred, specific responses—a cookbook approach to health, so to speak. Instead we decided to "chunk-up" and promote living a vibrant life from a position of homeostasis or balance. Illness, disease, and pain are symptoms of an imbalance within the body/mind, and once those are properly addressed, the symptoms diminish or disappear.

Research regarding health and nutrition is an ongoing process. In this book we discuss practical, proven ways of helping you live a vibrant life. Understanding and awareness are the key factors of any change. It is our hope that this small yet powerful book impacts your change. We were all born to live a vibrant life.

With love and joy!

Dawn and Robert King

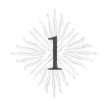

I Accept My Healthy Self

Accepting Your Healthy Birthright

You were born to enjoy "royal health" and to be totally healthy in every way—physically, mentally, emotionally, and spiritually. Your fantastic physical body is designed to be lean, strong, and flexible and to have amazing power and endurance. Your body, which is filled with unimaginable innate wisdom and the ability to grow and repair itself, is meant to be the home of powerful muscles, strong bones, healthy blood cells and circulation, fully functioning organs, and happy hormones.

Your marvelous mental body is designed to be clear, sharp, and highly creative. It was created with the ability to process huge amounts of data at lightning speed. It is also designed with the ability to provide you with a razor-sharp memory! It can show you the past, the present, and even the future. Even the most sophisticated computer can't hold a candle to your fantastic mental body.

Your emotional body is exquisite. In fact, human emotions are unique among planet earth's life forms! They allow us to experience a full range of feelings—from fear and anger to joyfulness and un-bridled passion (well, you want to be human, don't you?)—while constantly returning us to a place of natural, effortless balance which includes peace, love and joy. Our emotions can make life a pleasure and offer us motivation, inspiration, and commitment.

Your spiritual body is designed to provide an experience of real and constant connection with yourself and with a power greater than yourself. Every tradition in every age and in every corner of the world refers to this connection in some way or another.

You were born to live fully and completely and to enjoy life and all that it has to offer. You are meant to grow, thrive, and mature with grace and ease. Illness, disease, and pain are not part of that plan. You were born to experience life with all your senses and to embrace each of your days (and nights) with optimistic acceptance, energy, and happiness. Accept no substitutes. *You were made to live a vibrant life!*

A Road Less Traveled . . .
The Road to "Royal Health"

Almost everyone is born with the potential to live and enjoy a life of "royal health"! Royal health means that all four aspects of health—physical, mental, emotional, and spiritual—are performing optimally and *in balance* with each other. I know this is not everyone's current experience, but it can be!

If you could design your life (and you must!), would you create one that was dull, boring, depressed, stifled, disconnected, lonely, restricted, and painful? Would you design your life so that your constant companions could be illness, disease, overweight, tiredness, weakness, and stiffness? Of course not! Who would intentionally do that? Not me and not you! Who wants to catch a cold every time your neighbor sneezes, or be held hostage by every terrorist microbe on the planet because of an under-functioning, compromised immune system? Not me, and not you either! I want a life that has boundless energy and joyfulness, one that exudes flexibility and strength, one with amazing vitality, and so do you!

I Pick Porsche!

Now, I might not be able to design or choose my height or shoe size, but I do have the ability to completely control my lifestyle, my thoughts and feelings, my attitude and beliefs, and therefore my health! Look—if life were a car would you choose a crusty, rusty, cantankerous, broken-down old jalopy? Who would want a vehicle that is hard to start, difficult to steer, always breaking down and in need of repairs, powerless and slow, unattractive, uncomfortable, and uninspiring? Not me. I want my vehicle (my life and my health) to be like a Porsche—powerful, luxurious, appealing, sporty, inspiring, safe, reliable, imaginative, innovative, and committed to a world-class standard of excellence! I want a vehicle that has meticulous engineering and aerodynamic design, with attention to detail and enduring craftsmanship. I want a vehicle that starts without fail, performs flawlessly in every season, is well-mannered, and can purr like a kitten or roar like a lion and seize the moment when necessary—a vehicle with physical strength and flexibility, emotional vitality, and mental alertness and toughness. Now *that* is the healthy life I want!

We can design a life that is a joy to live! In fact, why design any other kind? It's simple. All that is necessary is to put some time and attention into each of the four aspects of health (physical, emotional, mental, and spiritual) on a regular, consistent basis, and we will enjoy an amazing, healthful life—a truly vibrant life!

Knee Bone Connected to the Thigh Bone

When clients come to me I usually have to educate them on some basics. Many of them do not realize that their mind and body are connected! They don't know that their thoughts, feelings, and emotions affect their physiology in meaningful and even profound ways, and vice versa. For example, many of them don't realize that what they eat and drink affects their physical body and how they feel. They don't get that their anger and their joy have huge (and very different) effects on their body. They have no insight into the fact that their beliefs shape their lives and their health. Instead they see things as disconnected, isolated, and separate. The truth is all the "parts" are connected electrically and chemically and cannot be separated.

Feelings, Oh Oh Oh Feelings . . .

Some people are just beginning to realize that their emotions and feelings have a huge effect on their physical health. Others are noticing how their emotions affect their ability to think and be creative, and vice versa. Here's the point—*all the aspects of health are important and they are all connected.* That means your physical body, and what you do to it, affects your emotions. How do you feel if you pump it full of sugar or alcohol? How do you feel if you don't give it adequate sleep or provide it with quality food on a regular basis? Many people feel really ornery and agitated if they miss a meal. If your heart rate is jumping and you're your blood pressure is thumping due to excessive caffeine or nicotine, how easy is it to feel calm, peaceful, loving, kind, creative, and centered? What happens to your vim and vigor if something has you feeling depressed or sad? It vanishes.

Do you know that when anger or fear get control, the body pumps out huge amounts of adrenaline and cortisol, which results in fast and shallow breathing, dilated pupils, increased heart rate, and higher blood pressure, to name some of the effects. Some motor skills (like running) are heightened but some of the ability to see, speak, and hear is diminished. Digestion and some other automatic processes are interrupted. Our body becomes more acidic. Feelings and emotions affect our physical body. They are connected!

Are You What You Eat?

Let's put aside the mental, emotional, and spiritual aspects for the moment and focus on physical health and the physical environment in which we live. Some of you may be old enough to remember that old slogan, "You are what you eat." Are you? From a physical health point of view that phrase has a lot of truth! However, in these modern times I would add, "You are what you eat and absorb."

Almost all of us are experiencing a lower standard of food and environmental quality, inside and out, whether we know it or not. This is happening locally, regionally, and globally. The air, soil, and water quality have suffered dramatically ever since the so-called industrial revolution. The past fifty years have seen an unprecedented assault on mother earth, taxing her resiliency to the max! Problems that did not even exist or were marginal, isolated concerns have become critical global issues in my lifetime. Global warming, greenhouse effects, major deforestation (how long do you think you could last with your lungs removed?), excessive pollution of every kind, and species extinction are a few that come to mind.

What does that mean to regular, everyday people like us? Here's how I look at it. We have a physical body that is made up of trillions of individual cells. For us to be physically healthy each of those cells needs to be healthy. In order to be healthy each of the cells requires regular, consistent high-quality nutrition, oxygen, and an efficient elimination system to remove the waste products of metabolism. The nutritional requirements of each of those cells include all the vitamins, minerals, and trace elements, and so on, regardless of the position on the food chain (i.e., predator or prey, meat-eaters or vegetarians). Traditionally these have been supplied by the soil in which the plants grow. Plant life, from the simplest uni-cellular organisms to the more complex multi-cellular organisms, are a critical part of the foundation of life on planet earth.

These days, however, we find the plants struggling for breath in poisoned skies. The rainwater and groundwaters which are meant to offer the plants life support from below are polluted and contaminated in many areas of the world. The soil is devoid of many of the minerals and the trace elements they once provided, and it cannot grow crops properly without massive chemical supports. These include fertilizers, pesticides, insecticides, and herbicides, all of which have invaded the food chain. So how can we keep ourselves healthy if the very foundation we rely upon for our cellular health needs is not able to provide us with the nutrients we need? We cannot trust the regular food supply as it offers very, very few nutritional benefits today. The "standard American diet" preferred by so many consumers worldwide makes matters even worse. What are we to do?

If Health Is Our Goal, We MUST Take Nutritional Supplements!

When we consider the amount of stress most people endure plus the destructive lifestyles so many people choose, the importance of high-quality nutritional supplementation and wise food choices to support our physical body has never been greater!

It is absolutely tragic to me that about 60 million children starve to death annually. In "developed countries" we have a different problem. We don't starve to death—instead we eat ourselves to death. But we don't get the nutrients vital to life because they are no longer available in the regular food supply. We are overfed but undernourished. But . . . I am an eternal optimist, and I believe there is still time to find a happy ending.

All Supplements Are Not Created Equally

If there is only one thing I would like you to get from reading this book, it is this: hope. My prayer for you is that you will truly know that there is hope for a better, happier, and healthier life for all of us and that there is still time. However, we will need to embrace some change for that to become a reality. This book is about how.

Question: Who needs to supplement their food plans with high-quality, natural nutrients?

Answer: In my opinion, everyone who has a body!

There are people who think supplements are unnecessary and a complete waste of time and money. (I suggest those are likely the same people who think acid rain is not a problem either!). Many indigenous cultures have practiced supplementation for eons. They added specifically selected foods from nature to fortify their staple diet. They likely just called it eating. However, supplementation is a relatively new field for many people. There is a lot of mis-information and many contradictory opinions around. It is up to you, as it was up to me, to educate yourself about nutrition and supplementation. I believe in self-responsibility. In the following chapters, I will talk lots more about nutritional supplements and about living an accountable life, but for now let me say this: I believe that nutritional supplements are unequivocally necessary for everyone's good health today.

Caveat Emptor

However, all supplements are not created equally and all companies that sell them are not created equally either. The workings of our bodies are extremely complex. We have come a long way in understanding these inner workings, but there are many mysteries that remain. I sometimes think of it this way: for thousands of years nature supplied all the things the body requires for life from the local food sources. Whether we lived in the tropical jungle, the frozen arctic, high in the mountains, or along the plains we obtained all the necessary nutrients from our foods, which were eaten whole. It's only in recent years that we have had the technology to isolate and then replicate various individual parts, such as vitamins and minerals. There are profound synergistic effects that are simply not available when things are taken in isolation. Therefore, search out supplements that are synergistically produced and come from organic whole food sources rather than isolated chemicals.

You will get the most benefits from premium, high-quality products made from natural, organic sources and distributed by reputable, ethical companies. Do your research. Check around, and ask lots of questions. Compare brands. There are lots of "old jalopies" out there. Don't settle for anything less than a Porsche! Check out the products offered by health food stores and by naturopaths. It may be surprising to some of you, but some of the finest and most effective nutrition supplements I've found are available from a few select network marketing companies.

Wakey, Wakey

When people ask who I am and what I do, I tell them, "I'm Dawn. I wake people up!" I want to share with you, in a simple and clear manner, information gleaned from more than forty years (combined between Robert and me) of study and work with clients.

I want to show you what royal health is and how to regain and improve yours! Please remember as we pull the components apart, that it is an artificial separation; all the parts go together to make the whole. Our amazing selves and royal health only exist in whole form.

Let's Get Physical

When I meet with clients initially I usually explain to them what I mean by physical health, so there is little room for misunderstanding. The "health bar" has been placed so low in the modern world that there is often confusion over what is "common" and what is "normal." I can tell you that what is common today is not normal, especially in North America. It's substandard! And, in my experience, what is normal is uncommon. We are *all* deserving of normal health—that is, royal, vibrant health!

Okay. Everybody stand up. If this is you, stay standing. If it's not you, sit down, but keep paying attention. With rare exceptions almost everyone should enjoy a body that offers the following features: enough strength to lift and hold its own body weight (such as doing ten real push-ups), the ability to easily bend sideways, backwards, and forward (such as touching your toes), the ability to perform a sustained aerobic activity for at least twenty minutes (such as running), healthy blood pressure and blood sugar levels and all other vital signs within medical guidelines, appropriate weight for size, an uncompromised immune system, naturally fresh breath, an active libido, and at least two healthy bowel movements per day.

In addition, a physically healthy body has freedom from the following: aches, soreness, fatigue, sluggishness, sleeplessness, low energy, weakness, nutritional deficiencies, weakened immunity, getting rundown, and any premature signs of aging. It includes freedom from addictions such as tobacco, alcohol, drugs, and sugar cravings. The skin, the largest organ of the body, is free from rashes, hives, pimples, acne, other skin eruptions, and fungal infections, to name just a few. *A lot of these "conditions" are signs and great messengers that more balance is needed in the mind and body.*

In a physically healthy body the digestive system processes food quickly and efficiently with no signs of heartburn, acid indigestion, hiatus hernia, or constipation. The circulatory system is unhampered, blood flows smoothly, and all the body extremities are appropriately warm. The resting heart rate is regular, slow, and strong, and blood pressure is within established limits. All organs—such as the pancreas, liver, and kidneys—perform their functions flawlessly. The endocrine system provides and delivers happy hormones for a regular and pain-free menstrual cycle and offers both men and women a robust libido and sexual function, as well as the myriad of other functions delegated to the endocrine system.

A healthy physical body does not require any regular medication. A person with a physically healthy body naturally sleeps well. They enjoy six to eight hours of rest and rejuvenation and awaken refreshed and ready to embrace a brand new day.

All of this becomes the *minimum* for a physically healthy body—royal health. I will cheer the day when more and more people who live a modern lifestyle can meet the minimum standards for royal health!

Okay. If you are still standing, your physical health is exceptional by today's standards, so give yourself a huge pat on the back!

I remember one of my clients who, during our initial meeting, asked me in all sincerity, "Dawn, I seem to get a lot of headaches. Do you think I might have an aspirin deficiency?"

"An aspirin deficiency! Are you kidding me?"

Boy, do we laugh about that one now!

I told him, "The good news is, in a relatively short period of time, it is possible for most people to achieve this worthy ideal of royal health—especially you!"

The Executive Summary

Is your life very fast-paced and are you in a hurry and really busy
—maybe too busy?! Let me cut to the chase and give you the
executive summary.

Here it is—the three E's, especially for executives:

+ EAT right,
+ EXERCISE right,
+ ELIMINATE right.

Do this and you will be on the royal road to a real executive
lifestyle! Don't do this and you will be on the way to fatigue,
low energy, free radical damage, sore muscles, aches, memory
dysfunction, and premature aging. You won't be able to do an
executive's job, because you won't have the strength, energy, or
stamina to establish and maintain an executive's role.

Eating right means eating as low as possible on the food chain,
eating organically grown whole foods whenever possible, eating
smaller amounts every few hours, eating live foods as much as
possible, chewing food properly, eating 60 to 80% alkalizing foods,
and eating with peacefulness and joyfulness as your ever-present
companions.

I was grocery shopping with a friend recently. She chose some
regular, commercially produced, lifeless-looking broccoli. The
broccoli I selected from the organic section was full of deep rich
colors and fragrance. She asked me why I would pay a whopping
75 cents per kg more (about 30 cents per pound) just to have
organic. I eagerly shared that my organic broccoli is full of antioxidants, vitamins, minerals, enzymes, and trace elements. My
broccoli is rich in isothiocyanates—chemicals shown to stimulate
the body's production of its own cancer-fighting substances,
called "phase two enzymes." And best of all, my broccoli tastes

great raw or lightly steamed. Yours has almost none of that, but it does have pesticides, herbicides, insecticides, preservatives, and it tastes almost as good as styrofoam. My organic greens fuel and power my body and strengthen my immune system. Your greens offer a little fiber. Look, quality doesn't cost—it pays! Organically grown foods are where it's at!

Eating right means the elimination and avoidance of life-sucking, health-crippling, killer items that masquerade as food and drink. The power and influence of multimedia have now convinced at least the past two generations that it's "all about the taste!" Wrong. We have been duped! Just take a good look around at our nation's health and witness the pathetic, crippling, and unnecessary legacy of letting our taste buds override common sense.

C. Everett Koop, a former U.S. Surgeon General, has been quoted as saying, "Seventy percent of all North Americans are dying from diseases directly related to their eating habits." Yikes! Forty years ago junk gunk was a "treat" we might have consumed a little of once every month or two—a special treat at the Dairy Palace, or real homemade fish and chips at the Moby Dyck Diner. Now, sadly, for millions and millions of people it's a daily lifestyle, or more accurately, a "deathstyle."

According to the National Center for Health Statistics, in a typical room of 100 "average" adults (50/50 male/female, 25+ years of age) in America today, you will find (approximately):

+ 50 or more people are overweight
+ 33 people are considered obese
+ Half the men are at risk for cancer
+ A third of the women are at risk for cancer
+ 50 of the women will have heart disease
+ 25 people have high blood pressure

✦ 20 people have a cardiovascular disease
✦ 60 people experience a sleep problem a few nights a week
✦ 6 people have diabetes

These are only a few of the conditions that are influenced by the modern lifestyle. Most if not all of these conditions would be diminished or even disappear just by eating right. We must overcome the dangerous notion that all that counts is happy taste buds, serving convenience, and shelf life.

Today eating right means supplementing your nutrition plan with vitamins, herbs, proteins, essential fatty acids, phytochemicals, antioxidants, enzymes, and minerals made with the highest possible quality! Most regularly produced foods available today do not offer what the body requires. Planet earth does not currently offer the same natural qualities our ancestors enjoyed. Therefore we must supplement our diets.

Exercising right means engaging in aerobic activities that last a minimum of 30 to 60 minutes at least five times a week so that you break into a full sweat. It means doing activities regularly that increase strength and flexibility, such as weight training, Pilates, yoga, tai chi, and so on. Exercising means moving your body at any activity you enjoy that gets your butt off the couch: walk, run, bike, swim, dance, bowl, ski, martial arts, skate—whatever! Get moving. Do it alone if your life needs some solitude for balance. Do it with someone if your life needs companionship and fellowship for balance. For you busy "executive types," frequent, regular aerobic exercise is a must! Put it in your daytimer, Palm Pilot, Blackberry, or tie a string around your finger, but *do it!* Go sweat! Your life will work better on every level!

Eliminating right means regular and frequent detoxification and cleansing. In my work with clients (and with my own health care), this is the place I often start. After twenty years of experience with thousands of clients, *I am totally convinced that every body needs and benefits from regular cleansing.* Personally, I do a colon cleansing program a minimum of twice a year. Eliminating right also means regular bowel movements—at least two a day— big, plump, light brown floaters that are dispatched quickly and with no residual sludge.

Become a "pooper snooper." Pay attention to your eliminations. Healthy, balanced urine does not have a strong odor. Very loose stools or very hard, dry, compacted stools are good information for you about your body/mind. Things are not ideal. Hint: Most people do not drink anywhere near enough water on a daily basis! I know you will look forward to learning more about digestion in Chapter 5!

Eliminating right also includes regular sweating, as I mentioned earlier — not glowing, not perspiring, but full-out sweating! Most of the world's population lives in highly toxic environments and it is vital to our survival that we rid the body of these life-sucking toxins and poisons that surround us and permeate the air, water, soil, and most of our foods. We must flush them out of the body regularly and frequently. Personally, I like to break into a full sweat for at least half an hour every day.

Remember, however, if you are currently a medal contender in the CPO (couch potato Olympics), please consult your health support team before launching into a full-out assault! I have lost count of the number of clients who have come to see me because they were in pain from trying to do too much exercise too soon. Remember to start slowly and allow yourself time to build up your speed and endurance. And after the workout, be sure to replenish the water and minerals that were just sweated out!

Health and fitness are lifetime goals. If you have let yours slip for twenty years, please do not attempt to get it back in a few days. Whatever your chosen activities are, allow yourself many weeks, if not months, to build up again. And be sure to provide yourself with this key ingredient—adequate rest.

When the physical body is working as it should, we can live a vibrant life! Life can be easier and more fulfilling. We naturally feel more joy, connection, energy, happiness, and peacefulness. We are more productive and focused.

When we live closest to our ideal weight, our self-esteem blooms. We feel stronger, more in control, and more capable. Our energy can be focused on our interests and passions, rather than split on pain management and emotional distress. When the physical body is healthy, all of life is better. Remember the three E's: eat, exercise, eliminate!

My Intention

My intention is to help change millions of lives for the better and to contribute to the healthy evolution of our planet and the people on it. My intention is to offer you a roadmap and a success system to assist you and the people with whom you have contact. I want to offer you hope. Remember, all the parts are important and everything counts. My belief, based on working with thousands of clients, tells me that *supplementation is absolutely essential today and can help everyone.*

Some of the buzzwords I see in the contemporary media suggest we need a "quantum leap" in thinking and a "new paradigm" in attitude and actions, in order for our personal, local, regional, and global health to improve. I agree. What has been happening isn't working. We must embrace change and we must take charge.

I have promised you a simple, non-technical, pragmatic, and practical approach. I want to offer you the key ideas that I live by.

Please consider the ideas set forth here and take some action of your own. Be a detective. Be curious. Suspend your doubts and disbeliefs for the time being. (You can always have them back later if you still want them).

Start with You

The first person to influence and change is YOU! When people around you notice positive changes in you they will naturally want to know what you did and how you did it. When *your* life becomes better—whether it is better weight management, increased energy, more peacefulness and joy, overcoming an illness, abundant creativity, and so on—people around you will notice! Then, as you find these things help your own health improve, offer the information and support to others. Nothing "sells" and influences others like your own personal experience. You become the way-shower, the example, and the leader in a stress-free, natural way! Make your story a compelling and inspiring one!

The Challenge of Contemporary Life

Most of us are bombarded by almost constant negativity. We often call it stress—the stress of modern living. In fact, stress is an important part of life. However, too much stress has a debilitating effect on health on every level. Stress has always been there. The difference today is in two major areas.

First, there is a lot more stress around (much of it self-chosen). Stress used to affect a smaller segment of the population. Today we have stress-related problems (illness, disease, and pain) showing up in almost every segment of the population—young and old, rich and poor, male and female. This is unprecedented.

Second, we are making very poor choices for dealing with stress. Typically we seem to handle stress by stuffing it inside instead of expressing and releasing it in healthy ways. Then we overindulge in things that have long-term negative effects on our lives: overeating, over-drinking, over-drugging, overworking, and over-everything! To make things even worse we are in a hurry and we want it *now*, with no sustained effort on our behalf. We don't want to feel any pains, which are little messenger-gifts to tell us we need to make changes or adjustments to our lives, and where to make those changes. We demand instant relief to our *symptoms* or pain, but we seem unaware or unwilling to take action to look after the *causes*. We are the "immediate gratification culture" in so many ways.

Stress can have a number of phases, which can often result in disease. The first phase of stress is "fight or flight" which occurs as a perception of danger or excitement. Adrenal hormones are released. When those hormonal levels stay high for too long, regardless of the reasons why, the adrenal glands begin to function poorly. Adrenal exhaustion is the next phase, and it occurs when the glands are no longer able to keep up with the requested supply. We know this as burnout. Inflammation, over-acidification, free radical damage, and a severely compromised immune system result. The next stage is inevitable — disease. Typically people experience disease as fatigue and autoimmune disorders. There is hope, and it is best realized with a willingness to embrace change. Think about it. What got you to where you are now isn't going to get you out of here.

Trance? What Trance?

When Robert was doing some hypnotherapy training his teacher would say to the class: "Getting your clients into a trance is not the problem ... the problem is getting them out of the one they are in when they arrive!" 3-2-1! It's time to wake up!

Across the globe we are seeing illness, disease, and pain that were once reserved for "old" people showing up in younger and younger people. Eight-year-old kids with ulcers! Kids with heart disease, obesity, anxiety disorders, and legions of adolescents on pharmaceuticals and antidepressants!

Oh, *that* trance . . . 3-2-1! It's time to wake up!

Screentime . . . What's Wrong with This Picture?

We have nations of kids (and adults) who spend more than five hours a day of leisure time in front of a screen (not counting movies, computers, games), whose nervous systems are overstimulated, who can't do two push-ups or run around the block without having to walk. Their overstimulated adrenals are further bashed by terrifying images, intense music, excessive action and violence on the screen. Then they add insult to injury as they inhale huge quantities of candy, soda pop, chips, pizza, cookies, and ice cream. The American dream is becoming a worldwide nightmare!

There are legions of well-meaning but terribly naïve or uninformed parents who haven't the time, energy, or parenting skills to get their little darlings to do anything without "motivating" them with junk gunk and crapola (or more screentime). I refuse to call it food, because most of it cannot support life. It's the same for almost all "fast foods." It's junk because I believe most of it has it has almost no nutritional value and it's gunk because it clogs up the system. It has no place in a vibrant life.

Oh, *that* trance . . . 3-2-1! You know . . .

Loving Ourselves

What I am promoting is self-responsibility, self-awareness, and self-care. At the end of the day each of us is responsible for our own health—not the doctors, not governments, not the health insurance people, not the people making and selling junk gunk and crapola, not even the nutritional supplement companies— we are. We must become aware of what promotes and enhances true health on every level, and what limits, demeans, and diminishes health. Then *we must love ourselves enough to take care of ourselves—for life.*

The good news in all of this is that each of us can change, refine, and redesign our lives so that we can live and experience a vibrant life! Our thoughts, beliefs, values, and attitudes define our lifestyle. There is so much information readily available today in terms of nutrition, lifestyle, mental and emotional health, that ignorance cannot be considered an excuse anymore. Now it is all about choice. Remember, all products are not created equally. I urge you to choose a vibrant life for yourself, your family, friends, and those you meet. Love yourself enough to choose health!

Chapter Summary

The key ideas to remember are:

1. The 3 E's: eat, exercise, and eliminate right!

2. It starts with *you*—be the leader and raise the health bar!

3. Junk gunk and crapola are *not* your friends. Get new, life-enhancing friends!

4. Self-responsibility is the *key*.

5. Monitor and limit screentime and get movin'!

6. Supplement with the highest quality products you can find.

7. Everything is connected and everything counts. Everything.

8. Love yourself enough to choose health.

9. 3-2-1... It's time to wake up!

2

I Am Honest with Myself

All it really takes for most people to be healthy is that magical moment of insight and inspiration when the "light comes on." They realize royal health is up to them and they need to take responsibility and action towards it. For most people it's totally do-able. Take stock and then take action. I call it the AHA factor— assessment, honesty, and action! That is one of my goals for this book—to help you with the AHA factor: *assess where you are in a deeply honest way, make a plan, and then take action!*

Let's Assess the Situation

Here's an exercise you might find useful and fun. Get some paper and a pen, and go to a place where you can be undisturbed for a few minutes.

In this exercise I want to focus mainly on the physical aspects of health. Just write down your answers to these few questions:

1. How fulfilled am I with my present level of health?

2. How energetic do I feel at the present time (low, moderate, high energy)?

3. If I am experiencing some symptoms what are they?

4. If I have no symptoms, how can I enhance my physical health even more?!

5. Why must I make changes and take new action steps?

6. What is one health goal must I focus on and achieve in the next one to three months?

7. What is one health goal I must focus on and achieve over the next year?

8. What positive beliefs do I have about making changes?

Honesty

The next step of the AHA factor is honesty. I know it is the most effective when I am completely honest with myself. When I do the AHA process I know that it is just about me and only for me. I resist the temptation to get out the "truth bat" and use it on others! In fact, I would say that the changes and improvements I desire, with respect to all aspects of my health, are in direct proportion to my willingness to be honest and then to take sustained action.

When I consider my health today and where I would like it to be, I ask myself a few important questions that I want to share with you. Here are some of them:

+ What is so great about my health habits that I cling to them and resist changing or letting them go?

+ Am I living the lifestyle I would want others I love to live, such as my child, or my spouse? (Am I walking the talk?)

+ What will be the short-, medium-, and long-term costs of not changing *now*?

+ What new action steps will I take now?

+ By taking action now, how will this move me closer to who I know I am and who I can be—the real me?

+ When I free myself of these symptoms how will my life improve and how will I feel?

+ How will my health habits lead and inspire others?

You may come up with some powerful questions of your own —and even more powerful, insightful answers! We must take the time to truly and honestly know what we want. We must really get a sense of how we will feel when we achieve it. Knowing what we want and then taking action towards our goals is the fuel of freedom. In fact, we are simply being who we were meant to be—and living with outstanding health, energy, and joy along the way!

Believing Is Seeing

You may also become aware of some old, limiting beliefs about yourself and your life as you go through this exercise. I hope so! Some of them are quite cleverly hidden. This may be a great time to discover them and let them go. Then replace them with honest and true beliefs that really represent your true desires and abilities now. *We want to foster and preserve beliefs that empower us and fill us with the sense of possibilities!* All of us have infinite potential. Use your beliefs and actions to free yourself, now!

Lights, Camera, ACTION!

Look, it's great to "take stock" of our lives and to have beliefs that are positive and in alignment with our purpose in life. Fantastic! However, a belief by itself is usually not enough—we must take action. Results come to us when we take action every day. Every small step taken is an essential building block, and each block builds on the previous block. Everything counts, even if your goal seems like a big stretch for you right now. Do you remember this old joke?

> *Question:* How do you eat an elephant?
>
> *Answer:* One mouthful at a time!

(Be sure to chew really well and to take some high-quality, full-spectrum digestive enzymes with that meal!)

"Boot Camp"

You don't eat the whole elephant in one meal! Just take little bites. It's like that for most change. Just take little steps regularly and consistently. Some people can make massive changes all at once that seem to stick, but most people find life goes smoother when the transitions are less dramatic. You know yourself. Do what works best for you. In any case, record and plot your progress over a number of weeks and months and you will see amazing growth worth celebrating!

A couple of years ago I felt I wanted to improve my strength and endurance—in fact, my overall level of fitness. So I joined a fitness group. But not just any old fitness group—it was like a boot camp! We met every morning at 5:30 A.M. and worked out for an hour. For the first two weeks Robert had to "push" me out of bed. I wasn't used to getting up at 5:00 A.M.! Even though I have been athletic all my life, the program really stretched me in every way. I ached in places I didn't know I had! In the first week I couldn't do ten push-ups in a row—I could barely do three. But in three weeks I could! By six weeks I was used to starting my day at 5:00 A.M. and I really liked it—and by then I could do 25 push-ups in a row!

About six months into the program I came home and absolutely amazed my 16-year-old son and a couple of his friends, all of whom were "jocks." I hopped down on the floor and did five one-armed push-ups! Their mouths just hung open, until one of them finally muttered, "Holy cow! How did you do that?!!"

"One day at a time. One push-up at a time. Little steps, regularly and very consistently."

"Mrs. King—you rock, man!"

You don't have to do push-ups or run marathons or go to a boot camp. But, if improved physical health is one of your goals, assess everything honestly, make a plan, and then get going!

Designing Your Future

Now, here comes a fun part—designing your future! Just before you begin this next section, I want you to review the description of royal health in Chapter 1 so that it is fresh in your mind. Done? Now, sit and relax. I'm going to invite you to close your eyes for a minute or so, so make sure you won't be disturbed. In the privacy and comfort of your own mind, picture yourself over the next year or so. Really imagine it, just as if you were watching yourself in a movie, with pictures, sounds, and feelings. Imagine your health the way you would like it to be. Really get a sense of it!

Now open your eyes and for three to five minutes write about your "future self." Imagine what you would look like one year from now—you living royal health! Ready? What would you be saying about yourself? What would it feel like in your renewed body? How would your changes inspire others? Have fun! Begin and write.

Fantastic! Now you have a picture where you are today, and where you want to be. I'm sure you are on the road of royal health! That is the simple method I use to inspire action for myself.

Action that Nourishes

Our bodies require nourishment all day long. I'm not a big fan of "mega pills" for that reason. Our bodies are not designed to handle mega-amounts of vitamins once a day. B vitamins are a case in point. It's much better to take a smaller dosage several times throughout the day. Mega-dosages should only be considered for therapeutic reasons and are best taken with your health practitioner's guidance.

High-quality nutritional supplements are food and, along with healthy food choices, they will power our body's engine (cells) by providing consistent and regular nutrients and fuel. Now that's one easy, productive, positive action that you could start right now!

Hurting or Helping?

When it comes to taking action each and every day I ask one question: Is what I'm about to do part of the problem or part of the solution? Does this activity, food, or thought deplete me or does it give me energy? If it depletes me I do not indulge. Simple steps such as reducing coffee, increasing water intake, moving your body 30 minutes a day, and taking nourishing life-enhancing nutrients can make a significant change in one's health! You can count on it!

Plan Your Success

I have seen a lot of cupboards filled with dozens of vitamin, mineral, and herb bottles, but with no plan for their use—which ones, how many, and when to take them. Unfortunately those bottles often end up just taking up shelf space instead of improving the person's health. People are inclined to quit when there is no measurable improvement or results, but have they really followed a plan?

Sometimes I think of the body as a "team of systems" that knows how to act and interact in perfect order. We gain our best results when we provide those systems with nutrients in an orderly way. I am not a scientist in the usual sense of the word, so I am totally grateful that so much science and research has been done for us. We simply need to act on the information that is readily available. See the Executive Summary in Chapter 9 for some ideas.

Act as if your health and life depend on it—they do! As you use the AHA process you will discover how simple it is when you act upon it daily. You are building a muscle and a health habit! And with all things, the more action you take the more results you get to enjoy!

Actions That Get Results

Action (purposeful, passionate, and consistent) towards anything will produce rewards. If you take action towards your physical health it will improve—guaranteed! Of course you can use this idea in any facet of life. If a salesperson makes one more call a day, or generates one more lead a day, or makes one more presentation in a day, the rewards are inevitable. If a musician finds fifteen more minutes a day to practice, if an athlete finds a few more minutes to work out, or if a writer comes up with a few more ideas a day, their results will improve—it's guaranteed. Reading this book is a worthwhile action step. Congratulations! With each chapter that follows I will outline my steps and actions —they work for me and hundreds of thousands, so I know they can work for you!

During an initial consultation when I ask my new clients if they take supplements, many shake their heads. Those who do nod affirmatively often say they take (usually hit and miss) a super-market multivitamin or mega-pill. I tell them it's like trying to water a lawn with a thimble. It's too little and it rarely gets where it's needed most. The body requires nourishment all day long.

I tell them my #1 action step is to nourish my body with premium quality supplements daily, throughout the day. This includes vitamins, minerals, trace elements, herbs, multiple antioxidants, and amino acids from natural sources. I also like to include aloe vera and that amazing food, spirulina.

AHA! Just before you go ... what is the *one new action step* you can take daily that will give you vibrant health? Go for it. In the next chapter we will expand your awareness to an action step that will change your life and your health forever!

Chapter Summary

The key ideas to remember are:

1. AHA factor: assessment, honesty, *action*.

2. Taking action towards our goals is fuel for freedom.

3. Replace old, limiting beliefs with new ones that empower!

4. Take little steps regularly and very consistently.

5. The more action you take the more results you will get to enjoy!

6. I take premium quality nutritional supplements several times every day and I love to eat!

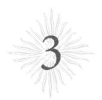

3

I Empower My Healthy Self

Acidity and Alkalinity

The relationship between acidity, alkalinity, and health is amazing, astounding, and even mind-boggling. Everyone who has a body or knows anyone else who has a body should know about acidity and alkalinity! This stuff should be taught to every kid (and parent) in every school every year!

Now, if you think this section might be a little too "technical" for you, why not give it a try and you may amaze yourself . . .

Almost anything can be tested to see if it is acidic or alkaline. We assign the term acid, neutral, or alkaline (or basic) based on where it falls on a scale called pH. Our body and the fluids it contains can also be checked for their pH levels. This is usually done by checking blood, saliva, or urine pH levels.

What is pH?

The acid or basic strength of a substance may be expressed in terms of a number, called the pH. The pH scale expresses the concentration of hydrogen ions (and hydroxide ions). pH stands for the "potential of hydrogen." We use a scale to measure pH that ranges from 0 to 14. The middle of this scale is 7.0, and is considered neutral. A pH of less than 7.0 is considered acidic and a pH greater than 7.0 is called basic or alkaline.

Now this next point is very important. An increase or a decrease in pH of 1.0 is *huge*. For example, a change from 6.0 to 5.0 is a very large change in the acidity level of the solution. This is because a solution with a pH of 5.0 is *ten times* more acidic than a solution with a pH of 6.0. Along those same lines, a solution with a pH of 3.0 is a *thousand times* more acidic than a solution with a pH of 6.0. ($10 \times 10 \times 10 = 1,000$). Are you still with me? Fantastic!

Human blood should be between 7.35 and 7.45. Even a slightly acidic blood pH of 6.9 can induce coma and death. (Saliva and urine have a different optimum value, which is about 6.5 to 6.75). Our wonderful bodies offer us optimum health when the pH is just about 7.0 or slightly higher.

The pH level has profound effects on all body chemistry, and therefore on our health.

All regulatory mechanisms (including breathing, circulation, digestion, and hormonal production) serve the purpose of balancing pH, by removing the "bad stuff" (caustic metabolized acid residues) from body tissues without damaging living cells. If the pH deviates too far to the acid side or too far to the alkaline side, cells become poisoned by their own toxic waste and die. Just as acid rain can destroy a forest and alkaline wastes can pollute a lake, an imbalanced pH corrodes all body tissue. Think of what happens when you spill bleach or battery acid on your jeans! If left unchecked, *an imbalanced pH will interrupt all cellular activities and functions*, from the beating of your heart to the neural firing of your brain.

Over-acidity is one of the prime causes of an unhealthy biological terrain.

Remember in Chapter 1, we outlined the importance of a balanced life—physical, mental, emotional, and spiritual—for optimum health. *Our lifestyle has a huge impact on our pH.*

We Choose What We Eat

What we eat make an enormous difference to our pH. Some foods are alkalizing and some are acidifying. Do you know which is which? It's critical to your health that you do! For example, junk gunk and crapola are acidifying. We don't have to eat them. We could choose fresh organic fruits and veggies. We could choose some quality home baking with real life-supporting ingredients. We could choose something alkalizing!!! *If a healthy body is the goal, we must make alkalizing choices far more regularly.* It's great to see some progressive schools removing junk gunk vending machines and more mainstream supermarkets offering organic foods!

Think GREEN

I was looking for a plant-based protein supplement because I wanted to reduce saturated fats in my diet. In addition I wanted something that was easily digestible and provided almost all the vitamins and minerals I need daily. Mission accomplished! It's spirulina, an amazing supplement that offers the same amount of protein I would get in half a pound of steak plus the same amount of phyto-nutrients found in several servings of broccoli, tomatoes, spinach, and carrots. It is a wonderfully beneficial and alkalizing food and I like to take it every day, either in pill form or in the powdered form mixed in a drink.

The list of spirulina's benefits for the body goes on and on. It contains the highest ratio of essential amino acids in a natural, bio-available form when compared to peas, beans, spinach, soy, whey, or egg whites (USDA listings); its completely digestible proteins assure healthy hair, nails, and skin, and muscle strength; and it is naturally abundant in numerous B vitamins to support nerve and brain function. These are just some of the benefits of spirulina. It's a whole food.

The spirulina I prefer is grown in a controlled environment to ensure its quality and it is certified organic.

Yikes!

I still see many people make food choices for emotional reasons and convenience, however. Even in my beautiful little corner of the world (British Columbia, Canada), according to Statistics Canada more than 30% of Canadian children are overweight or obese!

I was intrigued recently with an article in our local newspaper which reported that, according to Dr. Tom Warshawski, head of Pediatrics, Kelowna General Hospital, and chairman of the Childhood Obesity Program, "The lifestyle we are teaching our children is launching them on a trajectory of ill health, illness, and early death. If the current epidemic of obesity continues unchecked we will be the first generation in centuries whose children can expect to die at an earlier age than their parents."

But it's not just the kids. The Canadian Heart and Stroke Foundation has reported that in the last decade baby boomers have increased their obesity from 19 to 30% and that less than 50% of women and men eat the daily recommended servings of fruits and vegetables. According to the 2003 World Health Organization report, one billion adults worldwide are overweight. Overeating is one of the main causes of health problems facing the modern world. Not only are we overweight, but poor-quality diets are often causing an unhealthy, acidic pH. Over-acidity and overweight are often found together and they make a deadly duo.

The SAD Café

The "standard American diet," also known as the SAD, is the diet that all too many North Americans and people on other continents make their own. Typically the products are highly processed and contain elevated amounts of fat, sugar, and artificial and synthetic ingredients. This diet is generally low in nutritional value and leads to poor health. We simply require more understanding and awareness about nutrition and alkalinity/acidity, and we need to make better choices.

If we looked at the lighter side of how we eat, we might laugh at ourselves.

"Who wants some burgers, fries, and gravy?"

"How about some southern fried chicken, fish and chips, and chicken fingers slathered in ketchup, extra cheese, and mayo?"

"Anybody for some sugar-coated donuts covered in whipped cream for dessert?"

"Would you like that order Texas-sized, son?"

"You betcha . . . and give me one of those big ol' colas, but make sure it's a diet cola . . . I'm tryin' to lose a few pounds!"

Can you spell "quadruple bypass surgery"? It is good to take ourselves less seriously and to learn to laugh at ourselves. However, there's not much that's funny about obesity, heart disease, or diabetes. We need to increase the awareness and understanding of the long-term implications of our current lifestyle on our health.

Holy Cola Batman

It takes 35 glasses of water to neutralize one can of cola because cola is 1,000 times more acidic than water! And that is not with just any old water—it must be alkalizing water. And the acidity is just one part of the issue—the cola drink also leaches minerals such as calcium from the bones, paving the way for joint and bone problems. I believe soft drinks and soda pop drinks are endangering the health of our children worldwide. If there are not enough ionic minerals in the diet to compensate, a build-up of acids in the cells will occur. Kidney, liver, bone and joint health, immune function, flexibility, excretion, elimination, and energy are all affected by pH balance.

Now, how many people do you see have a cola and then reach for a gallon of alkalizing water? I don't see any either.

An acidic balance will *decrease* the body's ability to absorb minerals and other nutrients, *decrease* the energy production in the cells, *decrease* the body's ability to repair damaged cells, and *decrease* its ability to properly rid the body of waste. That's a lot of decreasing! No wonder I felt so crummy when my body was too acidic. And even worse, in order to try to make myself feel physically and emotionally better, I kept putting things in that were more acidic (sugars, poor fats, junk gunk) and added fuel to the fire!

Having an optimal pH balance in the various fluids of the body optimizes intracellular metabolism, and enzyme, neurological, and energy functions.

The kidney and lymph system are constantly ridding the body of cellular metabolites in the form of waste products. The kidney recycles valuable minerals and keeps the homeostasis (a $50 word that simply means "balance") of the body in check. Excess acid is excreted through the kidneys and urine. The pH of the saliva is an important indicator of the mineral and electrolyte balance in the body. Salivary pH is important as this is where enzymes start the digestion process and the immune system starts working. They depend on a specific pH to perform optimally.

Fresh Breath!

It seems that everyone wants fresh breath and clean white teeth. Did you know that the body's pH has an effect on that too? Food particles and the film that often remains on and between teeth are usually oxidized compounds with a positive electronic charge and an acidic pH. Acids tend to damage tooth enamel. Most toothpaste and other dentifrices do not counteract these conditions because they are also positively charged and acidic. I use an all-natural dentifrice that is alkaline.

The Importance of Oxygen

Energy is what our health is all about! And where does the energy come from? It comes from our cells, which rely completely on a constant supply of oxygen. And what is the leading cause of the death of cells? A lack of oxygen. Think about it. You could go for weeks without food, and days without water, but only a few minutes without oxygen!

Our cells require oxygen to live. When the pH levels are in a more optimal range, nutrients are more accessible and uptake is greater (up to 10 to 20 times more oxygen!). In an alkaline environment, there is abundant oxygen available to cells. In an acidic environment the opposite is true. You see acidic fluids "push out" oxygen, the key to life. An over-acidic body is on the fast track to illness, disease, pain, and rapid aging!

Baby boomers are spending billions of dollars (of their children's inheritance) on products, equipment, and services to try to slow down or reverse the aging process. They seek to prolong life and minimize the effects of aging, support their immune system, and improve their mental and physical potential. *A more alkaline pH is the key!* Biochemists and leading physiologists have long known that the maintenance of a more alkaline pH is critical to cellular health and longevity.

The cells of the human body depend on a balanced acid/alkaline pH. If the pH of any fluid is abnormal, digestive enzymes are rendered inactive, and our food does not digest properly. Food-bound microorganisms such as yeast, bacteria, parasites, molds, viruses, etc. are liberated in the body, which puts stress on the immune system. They make the body more acidic. The blood must maintain a narrow pH range, for life or death can result. In order to maintain the critical correct blood pH, calcium may be borrowed from the bones, which may lead to weakened bones. Remember what I said earlier about soft drinks!

In addition enzymes play a huge role outside of digestion in other body actions and reactions called catalysis. In fact, catalysis is controlled by enzymes. Most of these enzymes have an optimum operating pH range of 6.0 to 8.0 and become ineffective outside this pH range.

Biological Terrain: A Healthy Connection

There are many factors that play a role in optimizing the chances for a healthy body. Biological terrain assessment (BTA) was developed by Claude Vincent, a French hydrologist and physiologist. According to biological terrain physiology on health and aging, the optimal range of the blood should be between pH 7.30 to 7.35. The urine should be between pH 6.5 to 6.80 and the saliva pH between 6.50 to 6.75. One of the main determining factors in a healthy biological terrain is pH. It is not uncommon for the average American to have a urine pH of 5.9 or so, which indicates that the body is too acidic (optimal is 6.5 to 6.80). Oxygen levels in the body are directly related to pH. *There are two factors that are ALWAYS present in an unhealthy biological terrain, no matter what else may be present. Those two factors are an acid pH and a lack of oxygen.*

Death Is Not an Option

Not too long ago a friend of Robert's was diagnosed with the "big C" and given 8 to 12 months to live. The best they could offer was pain management. His friend was devastated and so was his entire family. His wife told him death was not an option and they must look for alternative treatments. Thankfully they found some that they were willing to try. His friend completely changed his lifestyle and embraced a new one that included the 3 E's and 3 R's. His new health team helped him alkalize his body via cleansing, supplementing, and food choices so that the immune system could fight back. They offered a wholistic approach that included emotional and mental components. His situation was critical and fairly extreme, but he overcame. Today he is like a new man, with no sign of disease, and he (along with his family and many friends) now looks at health and lifestyle through different eyes. Awareness precedes change.

In general, to restore a healthy pH balance, the diet should consist of 80% alkaline-forming foods and 20% acid-forming foods. To maintain health (once it is completely re-established), the diet can be modified to 60% alkaline-forming foods and 40% acid-forming foods. Eliminate or greatly reduce things that are not life-enhancing!

Generally, alkaline-forming foods include most fruits, green vegetables, peas, beans, lentils, spices, herbs and seasonings, and seeds and nuts. Generally, acid-forming foods include meat, fish, poultry, eggs, grains, and legumes, plus all artificial items. Aim for an 80/20 balance. Alkaline foods are awesome to eat! They digest well and help provide absorbable nutrients, which I'll discuss further in Chapter 4.

It is your responsibility to learn about nutrition and lifestyle. You cannot rely on the people selling you things to tell you everything. They don't. Many food processing companies are not in business to look after your health, no matter what they say. You must educate yourself about nutrition. If I am the one buying it and I am the one consuming it, then it's up to me!

More Greens Please

I want to share with you another fantastic product which I take regularly. I call it "green food." It's a blend of green foods such as organic barley grass, organic wheatgrass, organic flax sprouts, organic cabbage, and other nutrients like beets, pineapple, green tea, parsley, and spinach. Look for a premium brand that includes vegetables and sea plants which are rich in natural enzymes, trace elements, antioxidants, phyto-nutrients, and amino acids. Green foods contain chlorophyll, shown to be cleansing and detoxifying in the digestive tract and colon. Chlorophyll acts as an anti-oxidant in the digestive tract, helping the body resist damage from harmful free radicals.

Green food also offers natural fiber and contains valuable proteins and fatty acids necessary for maintaining cell membranes and other important structures. My preference is one that contains sea vegetables such as dulse and kelp, which provide a rich source of minerals. Green food helps my body alkalize with maximum nourishment!

The Family Winds of Change

During the past several generations in North America there have been huge sociological shifts in the areas of family, lifestyle, nutrition, and the marketing/promotion activities of food conglomerates, to name a few. Junk gunk and crapola have become staples in the North American diet. They have become part of the social fabric. The sit-down family meal has almost gone the way of the dodo bird.

Recently one of our boys, who is 17, brought home a friend to join us for a family meal. As we sat around the table enjoying a wonderful, healthful meal and good companionship, she told us it was the first sit-down family meal she could ever remember. We couldn't believe it! In her family of five, they never sit together at the same table to eat a meal. Instead, some eat in front of the TV, others take something to their room, and still others grab something as they head out the door. How unfortunate!

North Americans now consume more meals out of the home than ever. But even if it is not popular, trendy, or fashionable, I like to eat clean and green. I like to eat at home the best, and I like to eat with my family sitting around the same table enjoying each other's company. I want my food to enhance the quality of my life, not just give my taste buds a three-second thrill.

All Jacked Up

The effects of drugs, alcohol, and other chemicals could be a book all by themselves! For our purposes, however, let's keep things simple. The popular substances most frequently used— such as coffee, cocoa, soft drinks, wine, beer, hard liquor, drugs (both medicinal and psychedelic), and tobacco—*are all acidic.* So, just in the area of acidity and alkalinity, these substances are not desirable or health-enhancing. (Herbicides, insecticides, and pesticides are also acidic, so if you eat foods grown with them, the foods are acidic too.) Alcohol is not your friend. Non-prescribed drugs are not your friend. Tobacco is not your friend. Period. The sooner you end your relationships with them the better!

Thoughts and Feelings

"Okay Dawn. Let's say I do all those things you talked about—eat really low on the food chain, eat organically, include spirulina and green food, eliminate acid-forming items, stick to an 80/20 formula, and exercise regularly. Is there more?"

Yes. First of all, way to go for all those positive changes! They are huge steps in a healthy direction. It is vital to our health that we alkalize our body. However, even if we eat "clean and green" and eliminate all the acid-forming substances, we still are not out of the acid/alkaline "woods" so to speak. Remember I mentioned earlier that our mind and body are connected? Well, *our thoughts and emotions also affect the acid/alkaline balance.* Therefore, strive for healthy, positive emotions and relationships. Be sure to be kind and loving to yourself first, and then to others.

If you lead a life that has a lot of stress, make absolutely sure you have positive ways to counteract that stress. Include some regular activities that are stress-reducing for you, such as walking, jogging, yoga, swimming, and so on. Movement is good and so is quiet time. Learn to be still. Strive for the balance. Change any long-held negative thought patterns and habits you might have. (Just ask your kids or your family—they'll tell you exactly what they are!)

The Three R's

Remember the 3 E's? Now we will add the 3 R's. (No, they aren't reading, 'riting, and 'rithmetic). The 3 R's go hand in hand with the 3 E's and they are:

+ Relax
+ Rejuvenate
+ Rebalance

Our bodies, minds, and emotions are constantly striving for balance (homeostasis). When we place performance demands on our systems we must provide them with the time and the resources to replenish. Be proactive! Remember, the best medicine is pre-ventative medicine! Eat, move, love, laugh, and relax your way to excellent health, and be sure to include premium, high-quality nutritional supplements.

Dawn's Green Path to Royal Health

I like to do the "Ten-Day Lean, Green, and Clean Plan" to really give my body a boost! This is what I do for ten days:

1. Take my nutritional supplements 3 to 6 times a day.

2. Add a green drink 2 to 3 times per day.

3. Eliminate soft drinks, coffee, alcohol, sugar, and white flour products. (Don't worry—there are other foods on the planet. You can do it!!) Include lots of fresh fruits and veggies.

4. Eat organically produced foods as often as possible.

5. Drink *lots* of water—more than 8 glasses a day.

6. Exercise every day at least five days a week for 30 to 60 minutes.

7. Make sure my meals are taken in a peaceful environment with no electronic interferences such as TV, computers, and cell phones.

At the end of ten days my body feels great! I like to stay as close to that nutritional plan as possible, each and every day. Try it. It's alkalizing and provides me with amazing stamina and vitality. It will do the same for you too!

Chapter Summary

1. Everything we chew and swallow affects our pH.

2. Over-acidity is one of the *prime* causes of an unhealthy biological terrain.

3. Improvement in rebalancing body systems will occur if the body is alkaline.

4. A slightly alkaline body is the key to awesome health.

5. A lack of oxygen is the #1 reason cells die and a primary cause of early aging.

6. Everything counts, including our thoughts and emotions.

7. Supplements do not cure, but they help the body heal and rebuild.

8. Cleanse and supplement!

9. Include the 3 E's and the 3 R's: relax, rejuvenate, rebalance.

4

I Am Grateful for My Healthy Self

My Immune System

Immunity! Isn't that what everyone on *Survivor* wants? It means total protection from being voted off the island! Or how about "diplomatic immunity"? Now there's a license for freedom! What about your immune system? Does it offer you the total protection and freedom it should? In these next pages I want to discuss a few things about this wonderful and complex system from a practical point of view.

The immune system is not one thing or one organ—it is a group or network of cells, tissues, and organs that work together. It includes everything from bone marrow to the lymphatic system, thymus gland, endocrine system, spleen, and even the skin. *We have a community for immunity!* When your body's immunity is healthy it has a better chance to support your defense system. It must be on the job every moment of every day, because just by being alive we are under constant "attack" one way or another. Every day we must battle air and water pollutants, nature's own creations (pollen, ragweed, dust, etc.), byproducts of industry, and internal and external stress.

The immune system is widespread throughout the body and it needs an excellent communication system. One of its main methods of communication is with "messenger molecules" called cytokines which are also known as growth factors. It is vital that these cytokines do their jobs without impediment. If we are healthy it is a sign the immune system is doing a great job.

Now, you may not know a leukocyte from a lymphocyte or an antibody from an antigen. That's okay. The big picture is simple— the higher your level of nutritional fitness, the better your immune system will function. When you are nutritionally deprived, immune cells and other important factors for immunity may not have the level of nutrients to operate effectively. This can lead to a feeling of being overly tired and a lack of energy. The plan I follow to keep my immune system in nutritional balance is this:

- ✦ Lead a healthy, active lifestyle (3 E's, 3 R's)
- ✦ Follow the acid/alkaline principles
- ✦ Calm my mind and direct my emotions
- ✦ Take premium-quality nutritional supplements

Digestive Blues

One common factor that can contribute to an immune system being out of balance is poor digestion. Many people experience irregular digestion from time to time. Bloating and gas, improper elimination, mild constipation, upset stomach, and mild indigestion are common—not normal, but common. When the digestion is poor it can put the immune system in a bind or a predicament. Here's how. The body, in its wisdom, makes digestion one of its top priorities. Digestive enzymes are required to do that job. (Other processes—including the immune system, energy production, and even brain function—all wait while the body digests food.) That means when the digestion is not working the way it should, the digestive system "borrows" energy from other sources, so to speak.

Enzymes for Digestion

When food enters the digestive tract it needs to be broken down into the smallest possible molecules for absorption. When digestion is complete simple sugars, amino acids, smaller fat and oil particles, minerals, and phyto-chemicals are absorbed as they should be. Undigested proteins, complex carbohydrates, and larger fat molecules, if not broken down during digestion, may confuse the immune system in the GI tract. The immune system may start to react to the particles as if they are foreign bodies. This is called an **allergic response**. *The immune system is most active in the digestive tract.* So it is of the utmost importance to break down the food to its smallest particles. As we age, processes such as the ability to make adequate digestive enzymes become less efficient. In Chapter 5 I'll talk more about the digestive system and how to keep yours in top shape!

Enzyme supplements help to break down and digest food, and this in turn helps to alleviate the stress placed on the digestive system as well as the immune system. I prefer to use a premium digestive enzyme that offers a full spectrum of enzymes. I want a product that breaks down fats, a variety of carbohydrates, and different types of proteins, and can function in the GI tract at various optimal pH's during the entire digestion process.

Premium-quality digestive supplements usually offer additional nutrients called probiotics which support a beneficial intestinal environment. These could include items such as bifidobacteria, lactobacillus acidophilus, and other "good" strains of flora that provide the best ecosystem for the GI tract and colon. When the GI tract is richly inhabited by naturally beneficial flora then other undesirable types of flora are not as likely to flourish. In addition, premium digestive enzymes help cleanse the blood, increase circulation, and decrease inflammation.

I believe everybody can improve their digestion and support their immune system by including digestive enzymes every time they eat.

Auntie Oxidant and "Uncle" Al Kaline

They are my favorite aunt and uncle! Researchers now consider oxidative damage to be one of the major insults to cellular structures. This includes free radical damage in the form of hydroxyl free radicals, superoxide free radicals, and peroxyl free radicals. They are responsible for insults to cellular membranes, the DNA itself, including damage to the cells lining blood vessels, damage to nerve and brain cells, and damage to liver, kidney, and colon cells.

Look for a premium broad-range antioxidant supplement with the highest ORP (oxygen reduction potential) available. My personal choice has an ORP of –750 mV, which means it has millions of electrons available to "anti-oxidize" various radicals.

How Sweet Is It?

Earlier I talked at some length about the absolute need for good nutrition and reduced sugar consumption. Today the use of sugar in food processing is pervasive and it is included in all kinds of products. *You must read food labels!* Here are some more reasons why:

+ Sugar has been proven to destroy the germ-killing ability of white blood cells for up to five hours after ingestion.

+ Sugar reduces the production of antibodies, proteins that combine with and inactivate foreign invaders in the body.

✦ Sugar interferes with the transport of vitamin C, one of the most important nutrients for all facets of immune function.

✦ Sugar causes mineral imbalances and sometimes allergic reactions, both of which weaken the immune system.

✦ Sugar neutralizes the action of essential fatty acids, thus making cells more permeable to invasion by allergens and microorganisms.

When there is more sugar available in the blood than is being utilized for cellular metabolism, the excess in the blood acts as an oxidant, damaging cells of vital organs, glands, tissues, and blood vessels. The sugars are included in a variety of forms (sugar, sucrose, glucose, dextrose, fructose, etc.). It appears we've become a nation of sugar addicts.

Some artificial sweeteners are more natural and safer than others, so select products carefully and use them in moderation. But remember—*all of them are acid-forming!* It is vital to become aware of your sugar intake and reduce it! Personally, I avoid all artificial sweeteners.

Feeling a Little Stressed Out?

"I've only got one nerve left, and you're standing on it!" I've heard that one a few times—in fact, I've said it myself! It just doesn't feel good to be stressed out. I'd rather feel peace, love, and joy.

Okay Dawn, I'm with you so far, but let's not get into that touchy-feely, peace, love, and joy stuff!

Peace, love, joy and fun are my favorites! But I digress. Let's look at stress from an immune system viewpoint . . .

What do stress and the emotions that can accompany stress such as fear, anger, and frustration actually do? Tons! For our purposes let's see how stress affects the adrenal glands, among other things. One of the main purposes of the adrenal glands is to help you deal with stress from every possible source (psychological, environmental, infectious, physical, and emotional) and survive. *The adrenal glands produce a number of different hormones that influence virtually all of the major processes in the body,* such as adrenaline and cortisone.

Adrenal hormones strongly affect the utilization of carbohydrates and fats, the conversion of fats and proteins into energy, the distribution of stored fat (especially around your waist and at the sides of your face), normal blood sugar regulation, and proper cardiovascular and gastrointestinal function. As mentioned earlier, adrenal stress can lead to burnout and disease. Proper adrenal function is paramount for healthy living and stress upsets it. So now, about that touchy-feely stuff . . .

Toxic Wasteland

Our bodies produce a variety of toxic wastes just through the process of our own metabolism. We have the mechanisms and pathways in place to handle the "normal load." These days, however, we get toxins from just about everywhere and in amounts that far exceed anything in history.

In 1990, the U.S. Environmental Protection Agency (EPA) estimated there were 70,000 chemicals commonly used in pesticides, foods, and prescription drugs. Today there are thousands and thousands more. The use of pesticides, insecticides, and herbicides to limit crop loss has skyrocketed over the past thirty years. In the U.S. alone over 4.5 billion pounds of pesticides are used annually! *The average person consumes one pound of these chemicals pesticides, herbicides, and toxins each year!* Toxins and other unwanted chemicals are in many levels of the food chain. In 2004 a study by the Environmental Working Group found more than 280 toxic chemicals and pollutants in umbilical cord blood they tested. Our systems were never designed to handle this overload of toxins.

What do you suppose happens to these acidic toxins if they are not eliminated? They are reabsorbed via the colon into the liver, put back into the circulatory system, and can be deposited into the tissues. Toxic chemicals are accumulating in our tissues faster than we can get them out! The net effect is increased stress on our immune systems. This can result in illness, pain, and disease!

Pucker Up!

In her lifetime the average modern woman inadvertently ingests four pounds of lipstick! Jeez Louise! Typically lipstick is made from petroleum-based waxes with ingredients that can be artificial and insoluble. The ingredients give lipstick its colour, shelf life, shape, luster, and so on. Remember, whatever you put on your skin is absorbed and ends up in your bloodstream, where the liver and other organs are forced to deal with it.

Sleepless in Seattle, Saskatoon, New York, Mexico City, Topeka . . .

Many people (over 50 million in the U.S. alone) do not sleep well for a variety of reasons. When we don't sleep well, or when we don't get enough sleep, all kinds of problems can arise. Sleep deprivation can, in fact, undermine all areas of your physical and mental health. It makes us more acidic. *A lack of sleep weakens the immune system, leaving us more susceptible to other diseases and disorders*. The importance of a good night's sleep cannot be overestimated! Here are some simple, easy, cheap (free?) things I like to do to help ensure a good night's rest.

Eat Right, Exercise Right, Eliminate Right!

Is this starting to sound familiar? In addition here are some things I do on a regular basis to help ensure a good night's rest: eat a light evening meal, reduce or eliminate intoxicants and stimulants in the evening, reduce or avoid any stressful activities and instead enjoy peaceful, relaxing activities in the evening . . . a walk at sunset, soothing music, a good book, positive conversations—peace, love and joy! When my health is royal, a good night's sleep is automatic!

My husband Robert and I have *very* active lifestyles in addition to our full family and professional lives. We are regular runners (Robert is currently training for his fourth marathon, and I am training for my first triathlon), play on a volleyball team, have a rock 'n roll band, and have three kids still at home. They are all fun activities (even the kids!) and they all take tremendous amounts of energy (especially the kids!). When people hire our band or when we put on our own events we have to be in top form every time! We know that is absolutely vital to support our immune systems in order to stay in top shape and to do the things that mean so much to us.

Because I never want to miss a day of this fantastic life, here are some of the things I do to keep myself in royal health:

1. 3 E's (eat right, exercise right, eliminate right) and supplement right!

2. Stay aware of my thoughts—beliefs, values, and attitudes—and keep them pro-health!

3. 3 R's: relax, rejuvenate, rebalance.

4. Honor my interests and passions by doing them regularly.

5. Keep my life in balance, which sometimes means saying "no."

Chapter Summary

The Tribal Council has spoken. These are key ideas to remember and act upon!

1. A strong, nutritionally supported immune system is the goal.

2. An alkaline diet is healthier for the body than an acid-producing diet.

3. Antioxidants help stop damage at the molecular and cellular level. Take broad-range, high-quality antioxidants.

4. Read food labels and eat *real* food.

5. Become aware of and reduce sugar consumption.

6. Reduce stress and do things that promote peacefulness and play!

7. Take a premium-quality digestive enzyme at mealtime.

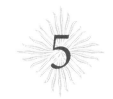

I Express My Healthy Self

Assimilate and Eliminate

When I look back on the last twenty years of my life they seem to have gone by so quickly! Marriage, birth, death, children, moving, work, travel ... "the stuff of life!" Yet each year has been overflowing with wonderful experiences, learning, and growth.

In the early days of becoming aware of improving my own health I decided to give nutritional supplements a try, just like many others have done. Over coffee my friends and I talked about the benefits we hoped we would receive. We were impressed with the many testimonials we heard and read in the media. So with a heart full of optimism I went to the store and, as a prudent shopper, bought the cheapest stuff I could find. I took them for a couple of weeks, anticipating big changes in my well-being. Several weeks later, besides a change in the color of my urine, and a little less "jingle in my jeans," I noticed no differences. My optimism started to sag. My friends all had a similar experience. So much for supplements ... but wait!

Healthy Steps

One glorious day, when I had all but dismissed the idea of supplementation, and was looking for some "inspiration for my constitution" I came upon a copy of a book called *Healthy Steps* by Dr. Albert Zehr. I tore through that book as fast as my eyes would go and my brain would comprehend! The book made complete and total sense to me. No wonder I didn't get the results I expected from those supplements! *I had made two fundamental and very common errors.*

The first mistake was to go to my local mega-store and buy the cheapest supplements I could find. Like many others I have spoken with since, I thought that all supplements were created equally, that one worked as well as another, and that the main consideration was the price. Wrong! The second "error" was my complete lack of information regarding cleansing. None of my friends or family had ever heard about cleansing either. When I asked them about cleansing they thought I meant taking a shower! I made it my business to find out as much as I could about proper supplementation and about cleansing, and I was going to be my own "test case." Dawn to the charge!

And what did I find out? I found out that *all supplements are not created equally!* It is of the utmost importance to use only the highest quality ingredients available. Premium products must be carefully manufactured using natural ingredients (preferably organic), and they must be combined using the most complete and current nutritional research so that they can "deliver the goods" where they are most needed—to each and every cell. I also found out that *all supplements are not the same and neither are the companies that sell them!* There are many areas where a company can take "shortcuts" and deliver less than is stated on the packaging.

The reason to supplement, I learned, is to *supply the body with more of the nutrients it requires in order to be healthy.* It's based on the idea that our current food sources (plus common food choices) do not supply enough essential nutrients in the first place, a most reasonable assumption in today's world. So, *supplements are a necessary addition to our food intake.* Then doesn't it make sense that the supplements should be as real as possible? Why would anyone want to take some chemically produced, artificial and synthetic substance to replace something missing that is supposed to be natural and real? I think of excellent nutritional supplementation as food.

My own health was not the best in those earlier days. My lifestyle included too many of the things that are not life-enhancing and not nearly enough of the things that are. I was an overweight and emotional young mom—the result of smoking, alcohol, junk food, stress, and no exercise. My skin was blotchy, my energy was low, and my moods were bouncing up and down faster than a two-year-old in a jolly jumper! I might have even been a tad difficult to live with . . . but I was eager to learn and willing to change.

Even though it seemed like a big stretch and I felt out of my comfort zone, I decided to begin my own "healthy steps" program right away. I found some nice people in my city who had the cleansing program available and I began that day. The people told me about another brilliant gem of a book: *Tissue Cleansing Through Bowel Management* by Dr. Bernard Jensen.

I read and studied and cleansed. Boy, did I cleanse! I became a pooper snooper supreme, and what came out of me was absolutely fascinating—kind of gross at times, but fascinating! At the end of the two-week program I took stock. *My energy had improved, my moods were more even, I had lost some weight, my skin was clearer, and my eyes were brighter. Best of all, I felt better!* My optimism was beginning to return. For the next two weeks I was mindful of what I ate and drank and, of course, I supplemented. I figured if one cleanse program was good, two would be even better, so after two weeks of "regular eating" I did my second colon cleanse program.

The second was even more dramatic than the first! It felt like years of compromised lifestyle choices were being flushed away. The pooper snooper duty was even more amazing! By the end of the second program I really noticed huge differences with the way my body and emotions felt. I had stayed away from the "coffee club" girls and just talked to them on the phone. When we met in person their mouths just hung open, speechless. I had lost a noticeable amount of weight, my eyes were clear and bright, my skin glowed, and my attitude was great! Of course, the speechless part didn't last long—after all, they are the coffee club girls! *They couldn't believe the changes they saw, and they all wanted to know how I did it.* I was more than happy to oblige.

Those two books had a tremendous impact on my health and on my life, and I am eternally grateful to both authors for their amazing contributions!

Basic Needs

Just as the health of a forest depends on the health of each individual tree, the health of the body depends on the health of each individual cell. The basic building block of the body is the cell. As I mentioned in Chapter 1 there are trillions of cells in the body, all with the same undeniable needs. In order to function properly (if not they die) each and every cell must:

1. have nutrients
2. have oxygen
3. be able to eliminate their wastes

It's the 3 E's for each cell! For us to be truly healthy each of our cells must be healthy! I think we need to let go of the current popular idea of "live to eat" and replace it with "eat to live."

A Chain of Events

The main focus of this chapter is assimilation and elimination. However, before we assimilate or eliminate anything, let's back up a little to the starting point. *Digestion is a chain of events that begins before we put food in our mouths.* The smell and sight and even just the thought of food can be enough to get things going—salivation occurs and enzymes are released. Most of us are aware of only a small part of the process of digestion—you know: chewing, swallowing, and eventually some elimination of wastes. What usually concerns us the most is the taste and appeal of the food, and the feeling of satisfaction after eating food. In addition, the potential for positive social interaction and connection are important aspects of sharing food. However, what occurs after the food is swallowed and out of our sight and awareness is critical to our health. The actual process of digestion is quite complex and well beyond the scope of this book. While it may not be so important to understand the science of digestion, it is really helpful to understand some basics.

Down the Hatch

Our marvelous digestive system is a series of hollow organs joined in a long, twisting tube from the mouth to the anus. Inside this tube is a lining called the mucosa. In the mouth, stomach, and small intestine, the mucosa contains tiny glands that produce juices to help digest food.

Digestion itself is a complex process, so here is the simplified version. Food and liquid are broken down into their smallest parts so that the body can use them to build and nourish cells and to provide energy. If the chewing is really complete then the alkaline juices in the mouth will almost entirely digest the carbohydrates right there! After we have chewed and swallowed, the food enters the stomach, which has three mechanical tasks to do.

First, the stomach must store the swallowed food and liquid. This requires the muscle of the upper part of the stomach to relax and accept large volumes of swallowed material. For optimum digestion to occur we must learn to work with the stomach and stop treating it like a garburator. It is very hard on the stomach and the rest of the body when we load (or overload) it up with all manner of food and beverages. I've heard many people tell me that they can eat anything and it doesn't matter. It's closer to the truth that they simply are unaware of how taxing that type of behavior is—the body and the digestive system know how much work it is even if you don't!

The second job is to mix up the food, liquid, and digestive juices produced by the stomach *and churn the food into pulp.* The stomach works something like your washing machine. This churning action is critical to the stomach producing the acidic digestive juices that digest proteins, which are long chains of amino acids (think freight train). Both the under-secretion and the over-secretion of digestive enzymes can lead to digestive difficulties. If the stomach doesn't churn properly, then sufficient digestive juices are not produced, making it difficult for the body to absorb proteins and vital minerals, such as calcium. The amount of difficulty with just these two factors alone would keep the Maytag Man running off his feet and lonely no more!

The lower part of the stomach mixes these materials by its muscle action. *The third task of the stomach is to empty its contents slowly into the small intestine.* The stomach activates vitamin B12 from our diet and secretes hydrochloric acid to break down food. *Substances such as alcohol, aspirin, and caffeine are absorbed directly by the stomach.* The stomach is susceptible to an increase in the concentration of hydrochloric acid brought on by stress, certain foods, and the effects of tobacco smoke. This disturbs and impairs proper digestion.

Two solid organs, the liver and the pancreas, along with the gallbladder, produce digestive juices that reach the intestine through small tubes. In addition, parts of other organ systems (for instance, nerves and blood) play a major role in the digestive system. The digestion of carbohydrates begins in the mouth and the digestion of proteins starts in the stomach. The stomach empties over a one- to two-hour period. However, *high-fat diets significantly increase this time period.* When the digestion is slowed down, the result can cause problems. Slow digestion may impact the body's ability to heal, so there are many benefits from a normal and complete digestion. *These are powerful reasons to follow the 3 E's and to include a premium digestive enzyme with each meal.*

Aren't you glad you're learning all this?!! Hang in there ... the science class will be over soon!

What D'ya Mean, Small?!

The small intestine can be between six and eight metres (over 25 feet). How does all that fit in there?!! The answer is it's all coiled up. The small intestine breaks down the food mixture even more so your body can *absorb all the vitamins, minerals, proteins, carbohydrates, and fats.* This is where final digestion and absorption occur. Food has been broken down into particles small enough to pass into the small intestine. Sugars and amino acids go into the bloodstream via capillaries in each villus. Glycerol and fatty acids go into the lymphatic system. Absorption is an active transport, requiring cellular energy.

Health Benefits of Aloe

What does aloe juice have to do with digestion? It can be very beneficial. Many people are familiar with aloe as a topical treatment for minor burns, sores, bites, and other skin irritations. Aloe vera is all that and more. Aloe juice, which is made from the leaves of the aloe plant, has properties that support the immune system. The active ingredients are the gel polysaccharides, particularly the acetylated mannans. Reports continue to reveal the healing properties of these plant compounds, and I am particularly impressed with the work of Dr. Clinton Howard.

Aloe barbadensis (commonly known as aloe vera) gel has been shown to decrease oxidative DNA damage. The aloe extract can also significantly inhibit super-oxide anion formation. This is one type of free radical that can have dangerous effects on the fragile DNA in our cells. Some users report an enhanced natural resistance to bacteria, parasites, and fungus (including candida albicans) with regular aloe use.

Aloe Vera Improves Digestion

Aloe juice has been used for centuries to soothe the stomach and related gastrointestinal upset. Some of the benefits users report include reduced symptoms of candida albicans, reduced bloating after meals, reduced flatulence, and improved elimination. Aloe vera juice may also act as a naturally mild drink for indigestion and can be taken alone or with meals.

Premium Aloe Gel

All aloe gel drinks are not created equal. I pass on the ones that use large pulp filtration, high-temperature concentration, whole leaf process, are decolorized, or offer added enzymes.

I'm particular. I want a premium product that begins with prime grade, freshly harvested, certified organic aloe leaves, and is produced with the least amount of processing possible. You might have to "kiss a few frogs." There are many pretenders out there so be a very particular consumer!

The Vitamin E and C / Aloe Connection

Vitamin E, a fat-soluble vitamin, protects vitamin A and essential fatty acids from oxidation in the body cells and prevents breakdown of body tissues. According to recent USDA surveys, the intake of vitamin E by women 19 to 50 years of age averaged less than 90% of the recommended daily allowance (RDA). Men of the same age had intakes close to 100% of the RDA.

Vitamin E is poorly absorbed when taken alone unless it is taken with dietary fats. However, when a 400 mg capsule was taken with two ounces of a particular aloe drink in a clinical trial, its *bioavailability was improved by 1,100%.*

In addition, a recent clinical trial conducted at Scranton University by Dr. Joe Vinson has shown that aloe vera gel enhanced the bioavailability of vitamin C by 170%.

Remember, we are what we eat and are able to absorb!

Meanwhile, Back at the Colon . . .

Back to the process of digestion . . . The mixture, which is called chyme, leaves the small intestine, exiting via the ileo cecal valve. It enters the large intestine, which is also known as the colon or bowel. The large intestine, which is about five feet long or so, is made up of the colon, cecum, appendix, and rectum. The chyme in the large intestine is mainly indigestible residue and liquid. *Water, salts, and a few additional vitamins are absorbed here.*

"Friendly" bacteria in the large intestine produce *vitamins* (including vitamin K) that are absorbed. Some vitamins, however, such as B vitamins and regular vitamin C, are meant to be absorbed in the upper digestive tract. For that reason I do not prefer time-released pills. The rest is (hopefully) eliminated.

Many people believe that the #1 key to good health is proper digestion, and I count myself among those numbers. When the digestion works the way it was intended, our bodies perform in accordance with its marvelous design. When the digestion is slow or functioning poorly, all manner of unwanted consequences appear. In my experience, it is unusual to find someone with truly effective digestion. That is why I am such a big fan of digestive enzymes, cleansing, green foods, aloe gel drinks, and supplements.

Paste

This takes us back to the second common mistake I made in those early days and explains why I didn't get much of a result from my first attempt with supplementation. I ate a typical North American diet. Therefore I consumed a significant amount of processed foods, many of which were white flour–based. I loved Dr. Zehr's explanation in his book, *Healthy Steps*, which goes something like this. When you mix white flour and water you get paste (glue). Ask anyone who has tried to remove wallpaper— when you put paste on the walls of your house it sticks for a *long* time. That's why people use it. Many people with bowel difficulties have "pasted" the walls of their colon over the years of eating white flour products. This leaves a relatively small hole in the colon through which the chime and feces must attempt to pass. It is also very difficult for the body to pull the nutrients through that thick accumulation of material. It's like layer upon layer of sludge!

So, even if you eat well and take supplements, most of the

available nutrients cannot make their way through the paste/sludge barrier and instead pass right through and are just eliminated. Eureka! By the way, "pastry" is just a fancy foreign word for paste! Remember that next time the seductive aromas of the bakery lure you inside! Healthy people greatly reduce or completely eliminate all white flour products from their nutrition plan.

Fast Food Fair

Science fair! It can strike fear into the hearts of many young students—and excitement into others! The inevitable science fair project recently arrived at our house, accompanied with the "I don't know what to do it about" announcement from our fine arts–inclined daughter, Aja. We brainstormed for a few minutes and came up with this one: Aja decided to take two burgers (one with cheese and lettuce, and the other just the meat patty on the white flour bun) and fries from a very well-known fast food outlet and put them on a tray. On the tray were also a couple of slices of whole grain bread, a small assortment of organic veggies, and a deli meats "sub" sandwich made with whole wheat bun. She wanted to know what would happen to those items if they were left out uncovered and at room temperature for a week. There they sat.

Each day we all watched with great anticipation. By two days the bread was beginning to go moldy. After another two the veggies were beginning to rot. At the end of the week we had to toss out the bread and veggies, and the sub sandwich was starting to smell. Interestingly, the burgers and fries remained unchanged to the naked eye—no apparent decay, and no smell. The only change we could notice was the lettuce was beginning to shrink from dehydration. We were curious about the burgers so Aja decided to watch them for an extra week. At the end of two weeks, there was no smell from the burgers or the fries, and no other visible signs of decay. Talk about shelf life! We kept them on the counter for almost a month. Considering what happened to the whole grain bread and the veggies we wondered if there was *any* life in those burgers and fries at all.

The "Queen of Cleansing"

Flashback to my first "healthy steps" ... I was so amazed and pleased with the results of cleansing that I did two things. First, I promised myself to do the program myself two to four times a year, a promise I have kept since then! Around here I'm fondly known as the "Queen of Cleansing!" Second, I recommended cleansing to most of my clients. It's hard to lose weight if the digestion is sluggish. The body just tends to hold on to excess fluids, toxins, and fat. In my opinion, the benefits of cleansing are huge and available to almost everyone!

Friendly Colon Critters

Your body has over 100 trillion bacteria. The majority of them are in the colon, and most of them are necessary to sustain health. The presence of these beneficial bacteria in the intestines aids digestion, synthesizes vitamins, and inhibits the growth of disease-promoting pathogenic bacteria. These friendly bacteria are called "intestinal flora."

Here are some of the things they do to support our immune systems:

✦ Aid digestion of lactose and dairy products.

✦ Improve nutrient absorption.

✦ Help prevent vaginal and urinary tract infections.

✦ Prevent colonization of the intestine by pathogenic bacteria and yeast by protecting the integrity of the intestinal lining.

✦ Lessen side effects of antibiotic therapy.

✦ Inhibit growth of bacteria which produce nitrates (chemical also used in food processing) in the bowel. Nitrates are bowel-toxic.

✦ Help prevent production and absorption of toxins produced by disease-causing bacteria, which reduces the toxic load of the liver.

✦ Manufacture B complex vitamins.

✦ Help regulate peristalsis and bowel movements.

✦ Manufacture essential fatty acids.

✦ Increase the number of immune system cells.

✦ Break down bacterial toxins (bacterial toxins knock out immune system communication pathways).

✦ Protect from things like mercury, pesticides, radiation, and pollutants.

Hey, isn't that a list!! You may be wondering what kills friendly intestinal flora. Many researchers indicate that the list includes chemicals, oral contraceptives, steroids, sugar, and the most common cause—antibiotics. Not being specific, antibiotics kill not only their intended "victim" but also the "good" bacteria in the gut, leaving the territory wide open to the growth of the not-so-good bacteria, yeast, viruses, and parasites that were resistant to whatever was used.

Note: Antibiotics, when appropriately used, are important medical tools that can save lives.

So by now I'm sure you can see that a healthy digestive tract, from top to bottom, is essential for a healthy body! Get it clean, keep it clean, and offer your amazing digestive system all the support you can! It is the #1 ticket to your good health!

Chapter Summary

Action plan for a rejuvenating whole body cleanse!

1. Order a premium colon cleanse program. Do this cleanse at least two times per year (fall and spring or winter and summer).

2. Drink premium quality aloe gel during this cleanse (and every day of your life).

The key ideas to remember are:

1. All supplements are not the same and neither are the companies that sell them!

2. The health of the body depends on the health of each cell, and each cell must have the following: oxygen, nutrients, wastes removed.

3. Supplements are an essential addition to our food intake.

4. The stomach has three main jobs: accept foods and beverages, break it down, move it along.

5. The small intestine breaks down the food mixture even more so your body can absorb all the vitamins, minerals, proteins, carbohydrates, and fats.

6. Aloe gel drinks have powerful effects on digestion and on the immune system. Choose your aloe drink very carefully!

7. Water, salts, and some additional vitamins are absorbed in the large intestine.

8. The colon hosts billions of necessary, friendly bacteria which are adversely affected by chemicals, oral contraceptives, steroids, sugar, and antibiotics.

9. Cleanse with a premium colon program, and be a pooper snooper! Support the digestive and immune systems with aloe gel drink and the supplements mentioned in previous chapters.

6

I Balance My Healthy Self

Happy, Healthy Hormones

You've probably heard of men who say that for a certain few days a month just opening their mouths to speak could be hazardous to their health! Here is our best advice for what to say on those days:

> *Dangerous:* "Are you planning to eat that whole thing?"
> *Better:* "There are lots of tasty apples in the cooler . . ."
> *Safest:* "May I bring you a glass of wine with that?"

Then there are those who notice their partner's libido seems to have gone into retirement. When you hear or see the word "hormones," what comes to mind? Once we get past the stereotypical answers and all the jokes about hormones, your answer probably depends on your age and your gender.

Hormones mean one thing to a 12-year-old girl, something else to a 21-year-old man, and something totally different to a 55-year-old woman or a man of 75. In this chapter we'll take a brief look at the who, what, when, where, why, and how of hormones, and what to do to get them in balance and keep them that way.

I have worked with many clients who had hormonal concerns. In my experience, when the other parts of their health were royal—

excellent digestive, strong immune systems, and lots of exercise and rest—hormonal issues were greatly lessened or disappeared altogether.

Hormones . . . "W-5"

✦ Who?

Who has hormones? Absolutely everybody! But hormones can seem like a spouse—sometimes it feels like "ya can't live with 'em and ya can't live without 'em!" Hormones influence and are influenced by a huge range of circumstances: some physical, some emotional, and some mental.

✦ What?

A hormone is a chemical messenger. The word "hormone" is Greek and means "to set in motion," "to spur on," or "to excite." All multi-cellular organisms (that's us!) produce hormones, and hormones are produced by nearly every organ system and tissue type in the human body. In general, hormones are produced by the endocrine system.

The major glands that make up the endocrine system are the hypothalamus, pituitary, thyroid, parathyroid, adrenal, pineal body, and the reproductive glands, which include the ovaries and testes. The pancreas is also part of this hormone-secreting system (insulin), even though it is associated with the digestive system because it produces and secretes digestive enzymes. Although the endocrine glands are the body's main hormone producers, some non-endocrine organs—such as the brain, heart, lungs, kidneys, liver, thymus, skin, and placenta—also produce and release hormones. Hormones act as a catalyst for other chemical changes at the cellular level necessary for growth, development, and energy.

✦ When?

From conception to death the glands of the endocrine system and the hormones they release influence every cell, tissue, organ, and function of our bodies. The endocrine system is instrumental in regulating mood, growth and development, tissue function, and metabolism, as well as sexual function and reproductive processes throughout life. Hormones are on the job every second of every day.

✦ Where?

Hormones are vital and active throughout the body, in every nook and cranny. The endocrine system is intricately linked to the brain and the nervous system, making it one of the most complex systems in the body. The *pituitary gland,* sometimes known as our master gland, is located in the hypothalamus region of the midbrain. The pituitary gland makes hormones that control several other endocrine glands; it is influenced by emotions and even by the seasons.

Here are a few of the other major endocrine glands and their functions. The *thyroid,* located in the front part of the lower neck, produces the thyroid hormones which control the rate at which cells burn fuels from food to produce energy. Attached to the thyroid are four tiny glands that function together and are called the *parathyroids.* They release *parathyroid hormone,* which regulates the level of calcium in the blood with the help of *calcitonin,* which is produced in the thyroid.

The body has two triangular *adrenal glands,* one on top of each kidney. The adrenal glands have two parts, each of which produces a set of hormones and has a different function. The outer part, the *adrenal cortex,* produces hormones which influence or regulate salt and water balance in the body, the body's response to stress, metabolism, the immune system, and sexual development and function. The inner part, the *adrenal medulla*, produces adrenaline which increases blood pressure and heart rate when the body experiences stress.

The *pineal body*, also called the pineal gland, is located in the middle of the brain. It secretes *melatonin*, a hormone that may help regulate the wake/sleep cycle.

Sex hormones are located in the male's scrotum. Male gonads, or *testes*, secrete hormones called *androgens*, the most important of which is *testosterone*. Working with hormones from the pituitary gland, testosterone also supports the production of sperm by the testes.

The female gonads, or *ovaries,* produce eggs and secrete the female hormones *estrogen* and *progesterone*. Estrogen is involved in the development of female sexual features such as breast growth, the accumulation of body fat around the hips and thighs, and the growth spurt that occurs during puberty. Both estrogen and progesterone are also involved in pregnancy and the regulation of the menstrual cycle.

The *pancreas* is the producer of two important hormones, *insulin* and *glucagon*. They work together to maintain a steady level of glucose, or sugar, in the blood and to keep the body supplied with fuel to produce and maintain stores of energy.

✦ Why ?

Hormone actions vary widely to meet the need of our constantly changing bodies and the phases of life and development through which we pass. Hormones act like an off/on switch influencing the stimulation or inhibition of growth, as well as regulating metabolism and affecting the immune system. Hormones also control the reproductive cycle.

✦ How Many Are There?

A hundred years ago or so, scientists thought there were but a few hormones. Today more than 100 have been discovered. A few recently discovered hormones are commonly known as the "hunger hormones." It is believed the hunger hormones give the brain/body information about when to eat, how much to eat, and when to stop eating. I know that on a number of occasions my hunger hormones have been dysfunctional—sometimes for weeks! As for the other hormones, maybe you should ask Robert . . .

✦ How Do They Work?

How do they work? Ask a pre-menopausal woman going through mood swings and hot flashes and she may retort, "Not worth a darn!" Seriously, hormones are released directly into the bloodstream. From there they travel to their destination, called target cells. The target cell has a special receptor, like a lock and key, so that the target cell can only be activated by a specific type of hormone. Once the hormone and the target cell link up, the cell knows it is to begin a particular function within its walls. The target cell may be located very close to the location where the hormone is released, or it may be in a more distant part of the body.

Hormones usually work perfectly to meet the body's constant striving for balance. They can act very quickly. For example, when the adrenals release the hormone adrenaline in the classic "fight or flight" scenario, the effect is felt in a fraction of a second.

Usually, however, hormones work slowly and steadily doing their jobs over time. For example, imagine the goal is to keep the concentration of a certain chemical, such as testosterone, at a constant level for a certain period of time. The hormones work the way a thermostat works. Think of the heating system in your house. When a room's temperature drops, the thermostat responds by turning the heat on. The room returns to the ideal temperature and the heater turns off, keeping the conditions relatively constant. Most hormones are designed to work in a similar way.

Dawn's Big Picture of Balanced, Happy Hormones

I consider the human body awesome, fantastic, and wonderful! I feel the same way about the mental, emotional, and spiritual aspects of living. The design of how it all works and goes together is nothing short of exquisite and even miraculous. When a person has royal health and lives a truly vibrant life, the natural, normal, and necessary changes we experience, whether male or female, happen in an effortless manner. Is that your experience?

I have worked with many clients whose experience of changes (hormonal) in the phases of life was so opposite to that. When I described the "ideal" they must have thought I just dropped in from a neighboring planet! Remember, *what is normal is not always common, and what is common is not always normal.*

My approach to having happy, healthy hormones is simple and straightforward. I believe in the 3 E's (eat right, including supplements, exercise right, and eliminate right) and the 3 R's (relax, rejuvenate, rebalance). For me the goal is bring the body, mind, emotions, and spirit back into *balance.*

It seems to me we are created to experience constant changes, inner and outer, as we cycle through the various phases life has to offer. And all along the way we encounter signposts and markers that let us know where we are in our journey.

The goal is to build our bodies with optimal nutrition so our physical, emotional, and mental experience is the best it can be. Stiffness, soreness, and low energy are signals that something is out of balance and needs our attention. In our modern world the tendency is to silence the messenger. You have no doubt heard it:

"Got a pain? Take this pill!" We get rid of the pain and then we often neglect to take the rebalancing actions necessary to look after the source of the pain. Don't shoot the messenger—thank him!

I remember once hearing someone comparing it to a person who just got a new high-performance car. As he was charging down the road the oil gauge started flashing red. But instead of stopping, checking the oil, and topping it up, the driver took a hammer to the gauge! No more flashing red light. A few miles down the road, however, the engine seized up from lack of oil.

Cycles of Life

Virtually every female will experience a menstrual cycle. Although it is a clear signal of change, pain is not part of the design. It is a similar situation with menopause, or "men on pause," as Robert calls it. It is a signpost along the journey of life—a signal of a normal and natural change.

In my experience, people who experience hormonal difficulties also experience digestive and immune system issues. These people inevitably experienced emotional challenges and habitual thought patterns which were incongruent with royal health prior to those difficulties.

So many of them are "driven," and their lives lack fun, enough rest time, and the 3 E's and 3 R's. I also have seen a large number of people with the opposite experience — these people seem unclear, unfocused, and are looking for purpose and meaning in their lives. They seem stuck. The point is that from one end of the spectrum to the other, what gets missed is the experience of balance and then the hormones get out of balance too.

It is curious to me that so many people believe that modern life is stressful. Okay, let's say it is . . . what are you doing about it?! Drugs, alcohol, stimulants, eating for emotions, retail therapy, and overworking are not the solutions. They are, however, part of what makes modern life so stressful! Instead of adding fuel to the fire, why not do the things that minimize and eliminate stress, like the 3 E's plus the 3 R's . . .

Here Comes the Cavalry!

There are some natural things to do when hormones are running amuck, in addition to the ideas I've already mentioned. Look for the wild yam plant. It contains dioscorea. It's an extraordinary plant that has been used for centuries to promote health and longevity. The Chinese have traditionally used the yam to cleanse and purify the liver, to relax the muscles, and to aid digestion. Ayurvedic treatments, which trace back to ancient India, include the use of yam to enhance libido. Traditional uses of yam include settling the stomach, calming an overactive gastrointestinal tract, and easing urinary tract discomfort.

Dioscorea contains structured steroid compounds that are almost identical to the body's natural hormone precursors. Your body may be able to convert these precursor compounds in the liver to supply the adrenal glands with the necessary nutrients for production of DHEA (dehydroepiandrosterone) and other important hormones. These plant hormone precursors do not act like synthetic hormones, which can have dangerous side effects, but instead they supply the body with the raw materials needed to produce its own vital hormones.

Many women today have rediscovered the value of the ancient yam. It is commonly used to relieve the uncomfortable symptoms of both PMS and menopause. Other properties of this plant render it valuable for reducing the stiffness of joints.

The yam's impressive list of nutritional functions includes its ability to increase the flow of bile into the intestine. Because bile is critical to emulsify fats this action not only improves digestion, but it also helps to support liver health.

Remember, hormones are not produced properly without ionic minerals. Be sure to supplement with high-quality ionic minerals. Ionic minerals are the smallest possible molecular structure in liquid solution that can enter the cell wall and penetrate the blood/brain barrier. Because of their size they are absorbed and begin working immediately to improve health.

Chapter Summary

The key ideas to remember are:

1. Cleansing, excellent supplementation, an outstanding digestive system, and a powerful immune system are necessary for proper hormonal functioning.

2. Hormones are chemical messengers mainly produced by the endocrine system.

3. Every body has hormones.

4. Hormones are influenced by thoughts, emotions, and other factors as diverse as the weather and the seasons.

5. It is normal and natural to experience hormonal changes, and those changes should be effortless.

6. Hormones are involved in every aspect of life and living.

7. Lifestyle choices and habitual (negative) thought patterns and beliefs influence immune system and digestive difficulties, which in turn affect the endocrine system.

8. Ionic minerals are needed in order for hormones to be properly produced.

9. The wild yam offers widespread benefits.

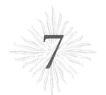

I Respect My Healthy Self

Nutrition and lifestyle are the foundation for physical health and development. Stronger immune systems, less illness, and better health result from living the 3 E's and the 3 R's. Healthy people are stronger and more productive, and healthy people of all ages learn better. Healthy people feel better and have higher self-esteem.

We have more access to knowledge and health information today than at any other time in history. We have sophisticated systems of information delivery. We have compelling reasons to get healthy and stay healthy. We have the technology. Why then, are there so many unwell people?

According to nearly every health-related group I could find, from the American Heart Association to the World Health Organization to the Canadian Diabetes Association, there is a big, dark cloud on the horizon. No, it's not my big fat Greek wedding, and no, Windex won't cure it! It's fat! Mountains of it. Overweight and obesity are expanding at alarming rates worldwide—regardless of age, gender, racial/ethnic origin, or socioeconomic status—and it is one the most compelling issues of our time. That means, worldwide, we are seeing more of the negative experiences that unhealthy people suffer and less of all the positive experiences that healthy people enjoy.

How Do You Know . . .

"Dawn, I've got some questions! What's the difference between overweight and obese? What is the line between fit and fat? Is 'a little chubby' overweight? Are skinny people healthier than regular or fat people? Are love handles okay? Can fat people go skinny-dipping?"

So many great questions!

Okay, here goes. Overweight refers to an excess of body weight compared to set standards. The set standards are guides. The excess weight may come from muscle, bone, fat, and/or body water. Obesity refers specifically to having an abnormally high proportion of body fat. One can be overweight without being obese, as in the example of a bodybuilder or other athlete who has a lot of muscle. However, many people who are overweight are also obese.

There are several popular and common methods used to arrive at these set "standards." One of them is called body mass index (BMI), and it can be used to measure both overweight and obesity in adults. It is the measurement of choice for many obesity researchers and other health professionals. BMI is a direct calculation based on height and weight, and it is not gender-specific. Most health organizations and published information on overweight and its associated risk factors use BMI to measure and define overweight and obesity. BMI does not directly measure percent of body fat, but it provides a more accurate measure of overweight and obesity than relying on weight alone.

The National Institutes of Health (USA) identify overweight as a BMI of 25 to 29.9 kg/m², and obesity as a BMI of 30 kg/m² or greater. However, overweight and obesity are not mutually exclusive, since obese persons are also overweight. Defining overweight as a BMI of 25 or greater is consistent with the recommendations of the World Health Organization and most other countries.

Weight-for-height charts are another measure used to determine if a person is overweight (although they do not measure body fat). These charts, which have been used by doctors and other health care workers for decades, usually give a range of acceptable weights for a person of a given height.

Other simpler methods for measuring body fat include skinfold thickness measurements and bioelectrical impedance analysis (BIA). In addition to body weight and height measurements, health professionals may also rely on a person's waist measurement to determine the location of excess body fat and the corresponding health risks. Analogous to BMI, health risks increase as waist circumference increases. A woman whose waist measures more than 35 inches and a man whose waist measures more than 40 inches may be at particular risk for developing health problems.

In my opinion royal health includes many things, one of which is an appropriate weight. Extra chins, beer bellies, pot bellies, and spare tires are not signs of royal health. I've heard it said that the average person today packs around about 15 to 20 pounds of unnecessary fat. That's like lugging around a case of beer everywhere you go! It's a lot of extra work for the body. If you had to hold that in your hands I bet you'd be motivated to get rid of it fast! Remember what I mentioned earlier about "normal" and "common"? We are seeing a greater percentage of overweight and obese people worldwide than at any other time in history. It is unmistakably more common, but it is not normal. One of the dangers, as we see more and more overweight and obese people, is that it becomes "the norm." As for love handles, I prefer them small . . .

Epidemic? What Epidemic?!

When Robert was a kid they had a little chant they used to tease kids who were overweight: "Fatty, fatty two by four, can't get through the bathroom door!" Like most teasing it lacked sensitivity and compassion, but Robert said they didn't get to say it much back then anyway. Oh my, how things have changed! *Globally there are over a billion overweight adults and 300 million of them are obese.* That is tons of fat, people! Obesity rates have expanded threefold or more since 1980 in some areas of North America, the United Kingdom, Eastern Europe, the Middle East, the Pacific Islands, Australasia and China. *Since 1991 the prevalence of obesity among American adults has increased 75%.* The obesity epidemic is not restricted to industrialized societies, however. Sadly, this increase is often faster in developing countries than in the developed world.

Oh, THAT Epidemic!

Obesity is a major contributor to the global burden of chronic disease and disability. In some ways obesity is a complex condition, with serious social and psychological dimensions. It often coexists in developing countries with malnutrition. We all need to work to turn this around.

Obesity and overweight pose a major risk for serious diet-related chronic diseases, including type 2 diabetes (85% of people with diabetes have type 2, and 90% of them are overweight or obese; since 1991 the number of adults diagnosed with diabetes has risen more than 60%!), cardiovascular disease, hypertension and stroke, and certain forms of cancer, especially the hormonally related and large-bowel cancers and gallbladder disease. The health consequences range from increased risk of premature death to serious chronic conditions that reduce the overall quality of life. Some of the non–life-threatening health problems associated with overweight and obesity include respiratory difficulties, chronic musculoskeletal problems, skin problems, and infertility.

Danger — #1 Killer Still on the Loose!

Cardiovascular disease (CVD) is still the American nation's #1 killer—claiming 927,448 lives in 2002. Cardiovascular diseases include high blood pressure, coronary heart disease (heart attack and angina), congestive heart failure, stroke, and congenital heart defects, among others. *Coronary heart disease is the single largest killer of Americans.* There were 494,382 coronary heart disease deaths in 2002, including 179,514 deaths from heart attack. In 2006, an estimated 700,000 Americans will have a coronary attack.

Overweight and obesity are major risk factors for CVD.

The American Heart Association's "Heart Disease and Stroke Statistics 2005 Update" included a new section on the metabolic syndrome (MetS). This information is from the Metabolic Syndrome Institute:

> The metabolic syndrome has been characterised in the United States in 1988 by G.M. Reaven. This adverse clustering of cardiovascular risk factors such as hypertension, glucose intolerance, high triglycerides, and low HDL-cholesterol concentrations was first proposed in the 1980s as the syndrome X. Subsequently, several other metabolic abnormalities have been associated with this syndrome, including obesity, microalbuminuria, and abnormalities in fibrinolysis and coagulation. Insulin resistance is thought to be the common denominator of the metabolic syndrome. Insulin-resistance is indeed a component of obesity, type 2 diabetes, and in many cases of hypertension, hypertriglyceridaemia with low levels of HDL-cholesterol.
>
> Obesity, and in particular the accumulation of central fat, also appears to play a key role in the pathophysiology

of metabolic disorders. Abdominal obesity, measured either by waist circumference or waist-to-hip ratio, is associated with insulin resistance and predicts the development of type 2 diabetes. In addition, abdominal obesity predicts subsequent coronary artery disease better than body mass index (BMI). Central fat accumulation and presence of insulin resistance have both been associated with a cluster of dyslipidaemic features, i.e., elevated plasma triglyceride level, an increase in very low-density lipoprotein (VLDL) and intermediate-density lipoprotein (IDL), presence of small, dense LDL particles, and a decrease in HDL-cholesterol.

The American Heart Association indicates that rates of controllable risk factors for cardiovascular diseases are increasing among America's young people. They reported that about one million 12- to 19-year-olds in the USA have MetS, with *the most common risk factor being overweight.*

The 2004 Canadian Community Health Survey collected information from over 35,000 respondents between January and December of 2004, and directly measured most respondents' height and weight. Canada's adult obesity rate was significantly lower than that in the United States, but alarming nonetheless! While 23% of Canadian adults were obese in 2004, the rate was nearly 30% south of their border.

Among young people, the biggest increases in obesity rates over the past 25 years occurred among adolescents aged 12 to 17, where the rate tripled from 3% to 9%. For adults, the most striking upturns occurred among people who were aged 25 to 34 and those who were 75 or older, where the rates more than doubled to 21% and 24% respectively. Though these rates may lag slightly behind their American counterparts, they still represent a staggering risk to the health of the individual and to the health of the nation.

The Problem Is Clear—What Are the Solutions?

I can already hear it: "Dawn, you are painting a pretty bleak picture here!" Yes, I agree, the picture isn't pretty, but it needs to be said. Awareness precedes change. I want to change your awareness so that you can help others change their awareness. Declining health, worldwide, is a huge concern, and it is changeable! Together we can make a positive difference.

Overfed and Undernourished

Most health-related agencies agree the obesity "epidemic" is, for the most part, due to two main factors. The first is an *unprecedented increase in the consumption of more energy-dense, nutrient-poor foods with high levels of sugar and saturated fats* (read junk gunk and crapola!). Coincidental with that is a decrease in the intake of natural, unprocessed fruits and veggies, and whole grains. The second factor is a *reduction in daily physical activity*, a result of automation and a sedentary lifestyle. I would add a third item: not drinking enough water. Fantastic positive changes can occur relatively quickly just by eating better, exercising more, and drinking lots more pure water! How hard can that be?!!

How Much TV Time Is Healthy?

Answer: If you asked Robert he'd likely say none or very, very little. The American Academy of Pediatrics recommends no TV for children under two years of age, and minimal amounts after that.

Part of the increase in the sedentary lifestyle is our love affair with the tube. As I mentioned in Chapter 1, estimates of average viewing time range from 2½ to 5½ hours per day for children and adults. That's for TV. It does not account for video or computer games or movies.

As far back as the mid-1990s reports such as the one featured in *Adolescent Medicine: State of the Art Reviews* (M. Morgan 1993; 4:607-622) state that increased *television use is documented to be a significant factor leading to obesity* and may lead to decreased school achievement as well. In addition, more than 90% of the "food products" advertised during breaks in cartoons and quizzes contain alarming levels of fat, salt, and sugar.

"People who spend a lot of time in front of the TV have this kind of couch potato syndrome," according to Dr. Frank Hu of the Harvard School of Public Health. "They eat more food … [consuming] more calories and junk food because of constant exposure to TV commercials. And they also exercise less." And, Hu said, they have increased risk of obesity and diabetes. *If you watch four hours of TV a day, the average for adults, you are increasing your risk of obesity by almost 50% and your risk of diabetes by nearly 30%.*

 ✦ People watching TV tend to snack more and those snacks are usually junk food.

 ✦ Kids in the U.S. see about 40,000 commercials a year. Sadly, under the age of 8 years, most children don't understand that commercials are for selling a product. Children 6 years and under are unable to distinguish program content from commercials, especially if their favorite character is promoting the product.

 ✦ TV personalities are often poor role models for healthy lifestyle choices.

Clearly, responsible TV viewing has many merits and there are some worthwhile programs available. It kind of reminds me of an ax or a hammer: both of them can be a used either as a tool or as a weapon of destruction. TV has the potential to be entertaining and educational. It is also one of the most influential mediums we have with respect to socialization, not to mention the subtle but profound power it has in shaping the beliefs, values, and attitudes of a culture and society. TV has played an immense role in shaping modern food preferences and lifestyles and in my opinion it has not been for the better.

The Skinny on Fats

Some years ago I enjoyed reading the book, *Fats That Heal, Fats That Kill,* by Udo Erasmus. It offers a comprehensive explanation of fats, oils, and lipids and how they work in the human body— which to enjoy and which to avoid. I recommend it.

The body requires essential fats for our very survival. I'm not talking about the fats found in donut shops or fast food outlets. I'm not talking about the stuff they slop on the popcorn at the movies or the grease they use to fry bacon and eggs and hash browns at your friendly local diner. Avoid those fats and oils! I'm talking about freshly pressed oils from nuts and seeds, such as sunflowers or flax seeds, and the naturally occurring fats found in plants, fish, meat, and some dairy products. I mean fats that are natural, complete, and preferably organic oils. Those provide energy-rich food/fuel to every cell, tissue, gland, and organ and are vital to many parts of our body, including our heart, arteries, reproductive system, brain, eyes, and nerves.

For example, fats are critical to the myelin sheath which covers axons, which are neural cells. Damage to the myelin sheath can result in all kinds of neurological difficulties.

There are fewer than 50 essential nutrients (about 20 minerals, 13 vitamins, plus a total of 11 amino acids for kids) that we must have and cannot live without. They are called essential because the body does not make them. We are meant to get them from our food sources. Two of those essential nutrients are called essential fatty acids or essential fats: linoleic acid (omega-6 or n-6) and alpha-linolenic acid (omega-3 or n-3).

The body is naturally designed to use fats and oils that are unsaturated and non-hydrogenated. However, processed foods and commercial food outlets offer exactly the opposite: saturated, hydrogenated fats and oils. Even worse, many processed foods contain trans fatty acids which are known to be carcinogenic. According to Dr. Joseph Debe, a U.S. chiropractor and board-certified nutritionist:

> Hydrogenation is a process whereby hydrogen gas is added to unsaturated plant oils under extreme heat and pressure in the presence of a metal catalyst. The purpose of this is to make the oil more solid at room temperature and to prolong the shelf life. Hydrogenation causes the oil to become more saturated and changes the shape of the fatty acid from what is called the "cis" to the "trans" configuration. These trans fatty acids are very destructive to the body. They interfere with essential fatty acid metabolism. They increase LDL cholesterol and lipo-protein (a) and decrease HDL, all of which contribute to heart disease. Trans fatty acids have also been associated with cancer, diabetes, immune deficiency, lowered testosterone in men, low birth weight in children, and impaired detoxification. Today's average diet supplies 2,000 times more trans fats than were consumed in 1850.

Our bodies are not equipped to process them in any quantity. Foods that contain hydrogenated vegetable oils and trans fatty acids include margarine, shortening, salad dressings, ice cream, fried foods, and most processed and baked goods, including crackers, chips, cookies, cake, and candy. Some European countries have banned trans fatty acids, but there are (currently) no restrictions in America. Food manufacturers have realized that consumers are learning of the dangers of partially hydrogenated vegetable oils and are therefore starting to omit "partially hydrogenated" and only use the words "vegetable oil" on labels of ingredients. Do your best to avoid all "vegetable oils" in prepared foods. They are *more* harmful than saturated fats.

© January 24, 1999 by Dr. Joseph A. Debé

Read the label! Avoid products that are refined and/or saturated. They contain little or no phyto-nutrients. Avoid hydrogenated products. Stay away from fried foods.

EFA'S

Essential fatty acids can help improve energy and stamina. I think of them as super foods that can aid in the delivery of oxygen and nutrients at a cellular level, optimize the oxygen-carrying hemoglobin and glandular functions, increase the metabolic rate and energy levels, and aid in recovery time of tired and fatigued muscles.

Another benefit of essential fatty acids is they help with weight management by decreasing cravings for junk foods, starches, and sweets. They make it harder for the body to make fat and easier for the body to burn it. Gotta like that!

Improve with DHA

DHA (docosahexaenoic acid) is an omega-3 fatty acid and an important building block of the brain tissue. *The brain is about 60% fat and DHA is about 30% of the brain* and an important component of the retina of the eye. It is essential for healthy brain and eye functioning.

Today the average American's diet is about 100 mg lower in DHA than it was 50 years ago largely because we eat fewer organ meats and eggs. In fact, North America has one of the lowest DHA levels in the world. Vegetarians are particularly vulnerable to low DHA levels. Low levels of DHA have been correlated with changes in disposition, memory loss, and visual and other neurological problems. This decline in DHA consumption has also led to an unhealthy imbalance between omega-3 fatty acids and the more plentiful omega-6 fatty acids. DHA is also important for maintaining a healthy heart and cardiovascular system. Fish is a food high in DHA because fish consume microalgae, which manufacture DHA. My preference is very high-quality omega-3 products made from organic plant sources.

Nursing Mothers

The importance of DHA can be seen clearly in the composition of human breast milk. DHA is the most abundant fatty acid in breast milk because it is essential for proper development of the baby's brain, eyes, and nervous system. Unfortunately, DHA levels in the breast milk of U.S. women are among the lowest in the world.

DHA is critically important for pregnant and nursing women. Studies show that breastfed babies who have an increased level of DHA in their brains also have IQ advantages over babies fed formula without DHA.

DHA for Healthy Kids of Every Age

The inclusion of DHA in a child's diet has been shown to improve learning ability, whereas DHA deficiencies are associated with both learning and behavioral disorders. Low DHA levels are associated with behavior problems in children and neurological conditions in adults. Mood disorders have been successfully corrected with omega-3 supplementation. Studies have shown that DHA can help improve difficulties breathing and environmental sensitivities. The positive effects of DHA supplementation are still being discovered as this exciting research continues.

Is Bigger Really Better?

I believe many people eat the SAD diet because:

1. They think it is more convenient and/or cheaper than cooking at home.

2. The fats and sugars taste great and make them feel good.

3. They think they are somehow invincible and immune from the ravaging effects of eating junk gunk.

4. They have lived under a palm tree on a deserted tropical island for the past 50 years and are genuinely ignorant and uninformed of the consequences.

You may have heard some of the rationalizations I've heard:

"Everyone else is doing the same thing!"
"Big is beautiful!"
"Bigger is better!"
"If I super-size it don't I get more bang for my buck? I'm just being a responsible consumer."

"Pizza is good for you!"

"I work hard—I deserve a treat."

That kind of marketing and thinking is providing the planet with short-term pleasures and long-term pains.

What's Being Done?

Did you know that the U.S. government now spends more money on education about the effects of overweight and obesity than on the effects of smoking? Governments in many corners of the world now recognize overweight and obesity as major health issues. It's safe to say that obesity is now considered to be a global epidemic. But it's not like Asian bird flu or HIV, or any other potential pandemic. It's not a virus or bacteria that you can "catch." With rare exceptions it's a result of dietary and lifestyle choices. I believe the most effective immunization against obesity is education and consistent supportive actions for ourselves, our families, and our communities.

Get Skinny? Not!

I think of obesity as an end result of behaviors. We see people digging their own graves one mouthful at a time with their knives, forks, spoons, and chopsticks. However, getting "skinny" is not the answer either. It is the polar opposite of obesity and too skinny is just as concerning as obesity. Anorexia and bulimia are eating disorders that can be life-threatening. The objective is excellent health and living a vibrant life. I have had some very skinny clients who looked great on the outside but were really unhealthy and out of balance on the inside. Skinny is not the answer. I don't think I can overemphasize this point—*the goal we seek is balance.*

There Is Only One You

Your body is unique. In this entire world there is only one you! It has its own amazing intelligence and it knows its own ideal weight and shape. It needs the opportunity and support to show you. There is no need for your body to look like or be compared to anyone else's body. None. Your body needs the 3 E's and 3 R's. Your job is to love it enough to give it the opportunity and support it needs and deserves.

Why Not Weight Loss Drugs or Other Alternatives?

Weight loss drugs, like all other drugs, are acidifying. That's a good reason in itself to avoid them. Some of the weight loss drugs work mainly by raising levels of the neurotransmitters serotonin and norepinephrine, which can increase metabolism and reduce appetite; others block the absorption of fat in the digestive tract. But many of these medications have potentially serious side effects, such as hypertension. Two drugs—dexfenfluramine and fenfluramine—were pulled from the market in 1997 after being linked to heart damage.

What about surgery? Look, if God wanted you to have a much, much smaller stomach, he would have equipped you with your own industrial-sized stapler. Instead of stomach stapling, why not consider a mouth zipper with a time-controlled lock? Or how about olfactory surgery to remove your sense of smell, or perhaps the surgical removal of most of your taste buds! You could opt for a tongue tattoo at the same time! Just kidding, of course.

Seriously, the best way to obtain and maintain your ideal weight is as simple as 1-2-3: the 3 E's and 3 R's, plus some high-quality nutritional support. Eat alkaline, drinks lots of water, turn off the TV, and move your body until it sweats—you'll reach the ideal weight for you!

Move It and Lose It

Imagine you're a car. You have a body. You have an engine. The engine uses a certain amount of fuel for the various necessary processes such as digestion, respiration, circulation, and so on. The more the motor runs and the body moves, the more fuel you use. You rest. You add fuel. If you add poor fuel, the motor doesn't work well. It sputters and coughs and misfires and has trouble starting. If you add more fuel than the motor burns, the fuel is stored in the body. It's called fat. Fat causes problems for the body and the motor. At the risk of sounding too simplistic, the formula is this: speed up the motor by moving your body frequently and regularly. Some people call it work and some call it exercise. I call it fun. Wanna lose weight? Burn more fuel. Put in less fuel than you burn, and make it good (clean and green) fuel. Rest. Drink lots and lots of water. The motor will take all it needs from the stored fuel (fat), and you will lose weight and feel better. Be the Porsche.

Action Steps to Take

1. Reassess your lifestyle and make small, consistent changes for improvement. (If you are just starting, seek advice from your health practitioner.)

2. Increase your water consumption with the eventual goal of a gallon per day.

3. Unplug your TV.

4. Instead of some artificial media body image standard, let your body be a reflection of your body's innate intelligence, and be happy with it! Imagine it, feel it, be it!

Chapter Summary

The key ideas to remember are:

1. Even though it is epidemic, obesity is not a disease. It is a result of lifestyle choices.

2. Eat foods rich in omega 3's and omega 6's and avoid the rest.

3. Many local, regional, and national actions have global implications.

4. Live with the 3 E's and 3 R's.

5. Remember, weight loss and weight management include eating healthy foods that are low in calories, fat, and sugar, and have a low glycemic index; plus a regular exercise program.

6. Move it to lose it! Shake your booty!

8

I Move My Healthy Self

Sports, Fitness, and Power!

A lean, green, energy machine is where it's at! Whether you are a world-class athlete, a weekend warrior, a slow-pitch slugger, or training for your first 10 km walk/run, you'll appreciate increased energy and endurance!

By now you know that the road to royal health and living a vibrant life mean regular daily movement, as much a part of your daily life as brushing your teeth! You know that your body was made to move—and how you choose to move is up to you. You know that every part of your life works better when you incorporate the 3 E's and 3 R's! You look and feel great physically, your emotions are strong, peaceful, and balanced, and your effortless and effective mental clarity provides fun and fulfillment. Let's see how to take our body's current performance and crank it up to the next level . . .

So Many Choices

Many people today have more leisure time than ever and they become involved in all manner of activities. For some it is traditional sports such as soccer, baseball, weight training, swimming, martial arts, and basketball. For others it is recreational activities like golf, curling, dancing, skiing, and hiking. Some people like spelunking or bird-watching. Others like horseback riding. Some of my Canadian friends enjoy snowmobiles in the winter and dirt biking the rest of the year. My Aussie friends like boogie boards and snorkeling.

The "Law of Increase"

Regardless of your chosen activities and passions, it seems to me that we usually want these two things at least: to have the energy and stamina to enjoy our activities, and to increase our level of performance, competency and enjoyment of them. *It is natural and normal for us to seek increase and growth in all we do.*

The Road to Royal Health and Increased Performance

The first step is to assess where you are today. If your current weight is too high and your level of fitness is too low, then start with baby steps.

Baby steps might include a visit to your health practitioner. Some people like to hire a personal trainer and a nutritionist as consultants. As you wish. The first step is to assess your current situation.

The second step is to make some short-term, easily achieved goals that can be reviewed weekly and even daily. Meeting or exceeding these goals builds confidence and helps keep you motivated until your new lifestyle becomes a "habit." (Experts say it takes about three weeks for most people to establish a new habit.) These goals may be recorded or charted daily and can be a visual record of daily food and supplementation choices, for example, or of daily physical activities.

Many people have found it helps to display a chart on their fridge or bathroom mirror. Two or three easily achieved goals are enough if you are just starting. Your goals can be about reducing your consumption of certain food items and increasing others. For example, your goal could be to reduce junk gunk and comfort food consumption and increase raw fruits and veggies on a daily basis. A physical goal might be to go for a 20- to 30-minute walk, or to walk upstairs and down instead of riding the elevator or escalator every day.

The key is to start where you are, have an achievable goal or two, and build from there. Remember "eating the elephant"? It's one mouthful at a time. In Asia they say "a journey of a thousand miles begins with a single step." Take that first small step. Success builds on success! *Start small and simple and then* KEEP GOING!

The third step is to reassess your progress regularly. For some people that will be monthly and for others it may be weekly. Reassess, and when the goal is achieved, *celebrate* your victory! Then make a new goal that adds a little bit to what you just accomplished. Go for it!

ICAN—Improvement, Constant and Never-ending

ICAN (of course I can!) means following the natural laws of increase. It means increasing or getting better or having more of whatever is important to you (not Häagen-Dazs!): physical health, great relationships, amazing creativity—whatever it is. I can hear some of you now saying, "But Dawn, if ICAN means improvement, constant and never-ending, does that mean I will never feel satisfied or happy about where I'm at with things? Does it mean my life will constantly change and I will have no sense of stability or security? Does it mean I will never feel good enough?" ("I think that is why I am overeating now!")

Relax. ICAN is a point of view in life. It's a perspective and a way of thinking. ICAN means I accept that it is natural for me to want the things that are important to me in life to be healthy and to grow and flourish—to increase and become more. All of life does that. I can feel happy and accepting about myself and my progress or journey in every moment. I love that T-shirt that says, BE PATIENT — GOD ISN'T FINISHED WITH ME YET!

There are No Mistakes

Recognize and celebrate each and every step along the way. Cherish your victories and be gentle on yourself if you backslide. Simply start over. One of my favorite authors is Tony Robbins, and he suggests there are *no mistakes—only feedback.* I like that approach. If my results are not what I want, it doesn't mean I failed. It means I haven't reached the goal yet, and I can see what I need to do to quickly get back on the path that is truly important and meaningful to me. *And* I can do it without remorse, recrimination, or guilt. I CAN!

ICAN does not imply reaching some huge, distant goal before feeling good about yourself. I want you to feel good about yourself right now! It also doesn't imply competition or winning a race. It does imply doing your best and having a more complete experience. It is about your relationship with you. Long-term goals are good too, in all aspects of life, but we must learn to love and appreciate the journey as well. We need to recognize and appreciate ourselves and have fun along the way!

Dawn, the Runner

Let me offer you a personal example of ICAN. When I met Robert he was a runner with many years of experience. I consider myself athletic but at that time I was overweight and a smoker. I was anything but a runner. When I visited him, at some point in the day he would say it was "run time." I wasn't able to run 10 or 15 km, so I would accompany him on a bicycle and we would chat the whole time. I was impressed with his level of fitness and even more with his motivation and commitment. Robert told me he really loved and preferred playing team sports like soccer and volleyball, but running suited his very busy schedule at the time because he could do it at his convenience. For that reason he usually ran alone. Without saying a word he inspired me to raise the health and fitness bar in my life. I decided to surprise him and do something good for me. The sports store staff was friendly and knowledgeable and they helped me choose a decent pair of runners for a "newbie." I was a strong runner in my earlier years, when I played softball and lacrosse, but I didn't have much experience with distance running.

Okay. Step one: assess where I am now. I'm overweight and short on aerobic power—I'm out of shape. But I don't have any other concerns. Step two: start small and slow and have a short-term goal. Okay, I want to run 10 km. Step three: after a short time reassess my progress. Right—sounds like a great plan to me!

One Small Step for Woman, A Giant Leap for Dawn

I remember the first run I did with Robert and his friend, David, who joined us that day. It was a beautiful spring afternoon. I laced up my new shoes and had a brand new water bottle with me. David and Robert were amazed that I was willing to tackle 10 km right off the bat. I told them I was ready for 10, even though I knew I felt rather nervous inside. Ah, bravado! We chatted about how good it was to be alive and set off really slowly on what was to be a beautiful 10 km run through the rolling rural hills on the outskirts of town. I lasted almost five minutes. I was coughing and hacking and spitting. My lungs felt on fire and my legs felt like lead. "You guys go ahead. I'll crawl back to the car and wait for you there . . . have a nice run . . ."

During the next few days my body talked to me about that experience more than it had talked in a long time—or was it just that I had not been a good listener before? It mentioned how it craved more oxygen, more good food, more regular movement so its joints and muscles could work without pain. My lungs and heart joined the discussion and they agreed. For them, they explained, the workload was becoming excessive. My body talked about all the additional work it was doing packing around this extra weight. It talked about strain it was feeling trying to digest the junk I was feeding it and how it was having a really hard time keeping the immune, digestive, and endocrine systems functional. It talked about the lack of water it was receiving on a daily basis and how hard it was to try to keep things going with so little support. It discussed trying to cope with no usable fuel. It explained it was having to borrow necessary minerals from other places and apologized for the pain that was going to cause. And it talked about how difficult life was on the inside when I was taking it for regular rides on the emotional roller coaster! And now you want to go for a 10 km run just like that! Are you nuts?! Okay, okay. I get it!

Back to the drawing board . . . Step one: assess where I am now. That's easy—same as before! Step two: start small and slow and have a short term goal. AHA! That was the feedback I needed and used. Okay. My goal is to walk 30 minutes every day at a brisk pace for a week. Second week, 30 minutes a day, alternate slow jog for one minute, walk for one or two minutes. Step three: reassess. Oh yeah . . . quit smoking!

I used that three-step process. I celebrated every day that I walked or walked/ran. I remember when I had progressed enough that I could run 2 km without stopping! Victory! It was like running the Boston Marathon to me! Ditto when I ran my first 5 km.

For me, a huge milestone was reached when I completed my first 10 km run. I wore that T-shirt like a flag! I celebrated myself. Over the year I had quit smoking, lost 25 pounds, increased my level of fitness, increased my self-esteem hugely, met some new friends for whom health and wellness were a high priority, and became an example and inspiration for others. I continued to use that three-step process with running and with many other areas of my life. To this day, it is one of the simple pleasures that Robert and I really enjoy—going for a run together.

Three Small Steps to More Success

Now, I am not suggesting that you need to become a runner. Running does not suit or appeal to everyone. I only used running as an example of ICAN and for using that simple three-step approach. You can *choose any activity that appeals to you.* If you are not sure what you might like, then go and try out a bunch of things. Go on your own or take a friend. Newcomers are almost always welcome, whether it's badminton, bowling, or ballroom dancing. You'll find something you like and meet new people too!

My suggestion is that you improve your level of fitness in every area of your life. Imagine being more physically, mentally, and emotionally fit than ever before! This mindset and approach may be used effectively by anyone, regardless of their current level of performance and achievement. My goal was to run more than four minutes without stopping. An elite runner may have a goal of reducing her 5 km time by four seconds per km! A bowler may want to improve their game by raising their average five points. Someone else may want to be able to touch their toes. What's your next goal?

Helping to Build a Strong Foundation

Once you have given yourself the gift of a foundation for good health by following the principles of the 3 E's and 3 R's, here are some ideas that will offer even more support.

MSM

MSM sulfur is found in plants, soils, fruits, and vegetables. Sulfur is one of the main components of the body and it is *critical for the flexibility and maintenance of cartilage, connective tissue, tendons, bones, and muscle.* Most people do not get enough.

Organic sulfur is necessary for making collagen, which is the primary constituent of cartilage and connective tissue in the joints. MSM (methyl sulfonyl methane) is a natural, organic form of sulfur that can be easily absorbed and utilized by the body. Athletes can benefit from taking MSM prior to physical activity because it tends to reduce painful joints, which may be associated with exercise.

MSM has been shown to encourage the repair of damaged skin. Our body creates new skin cells every day. *When sulfur is adequately available, the new skin appears softer and smoother.* The new skin cells are also more permeable, allowing toxins to be eliminated through the sweat glands, which relieves the liver and kidneys from their heavy workload.

MSM also crosses the blood/brain barrier so it can benefit the brain and vessels in the head and be helpful with relieving the symptoms of headaches.

MSM was first patented for its uses in the 1970s and one of its uses was for mild constipation. There is a great deal of evidence to support the use of MSM to promote regularity. MSM is a product that can be very helpful on many fronts!

Amino Acids

Amino acids are the molecular building blocks of protein and muscle tissue. *All the physiological processes relating to sport—energy, recovery, muscle/strength gains, fat loss—as well as mood and brain function, are critically linked to amino acids.* Anyone who wants to gain muscular strength must consume adequate protein or amino acids and exercise to build that muscle. This is true for a bodybuilder, a casual weightlifter, or someone who simply does not want to lose strength as they age.

Look for high-quality muscle-building amino acids in their simplest form, which are called crystalline amino acids. This means *amino acids are directly available*—they do not have to be digested.

When crystalline amino acids are taken they are absorbed fairly quickly (20 to 30 minutes) in the upper GI tract. As you exercise these amino acids go to the skeletal muscle, which means you can have greater strength and endurance to reach your workout goals. You will see greater muscle gains from each workout, and a reduction of unwanted body fat—not muscle mass—when you start a weight management program. Your recovery time will be reduced because your muscles are getting the fuel they need to quickly rebuild themselves.

Essential Amino Acids

Some amino acids are termed essential because the body cannot make them and relies on outside sources (food, supplements) to have them. One leading nutritional company's researchers have recently confirmed that there are nine essential amino acids, not just eight as earlier research indicated. The ninth essential amino acid, histidine, has been shown to enhance protein synthesis in the body. For great results look for a product that includes histidine as well as arginine and glutamine.

Energy Drinks

Here's my take on energy drinks and replacement drinks. I'm not a big fan of them unless you can find one that is ephedra-free. Ephedra is a stimulant and thermogenic but it can have undesirable side effects. Most sports energy drinks have sugar or artificial flavors, colors, or sweetener, and all are acidifying. Water is still my preferred drink.

However, it seems paradoxical that it is the athlete who most needs mineral replacement and supplementation. Why? Because couch potatoes don't usually sweat much. But athletes sweat, and when they do out goes water and minerals. That's why sweat tastes somewhat salty. Strenuous exercise is important and necessary for royal health, but it is acidifying to the body. That's why water, premium minerals, and rest are so important. Many of the popular replacement "ade" drinks use potassium chloride, which is a very weak electrolyte. I like to use a coral calcium and alkalizing water after sweating.

Speaking of Jacques Cousteau . . .

The ocean has provided us with the perfect blend of essential minerals locked inside its delicate coral reefs. These minerals are vital to the thousands of enzymatic reactions that take place in our bodies every day, so they can impact our health in an endless number of ways.

Sango coral calcium contains nature's perfect balance of minerals, similar to the composition of the human body. Sango coral calcium also enhances drinking water, and I like the ones that come in convenient sachets. One sachet added to 1 or 2 quarts or litres of drinking water will increase the alkalinity of your water, which is much healthier for the body. When added to water the sango coral calcium sachet releases highly absorbable bio-available ions to increase alkalinity. It also converts chlorine to a safer form, helps keep the body hydrated, and reduces oxidized free radicals. The sango coral calcium I prefer can be mixed with any noncarbonated liquid.

By the way, strict guidelines are in place to protect the environmental safety of living coral and coral reefs.

Premium marine coral is free of heavy metals and contaminants, giving us a completely pure mineral supplement. Be sure to choose sango coral calcium that is genuine coral, not limestone.

The Vitamin/Mineral Connection

Two-time Nobel Prize winner Dr. Linus Pauling said, "You can trace every sickness, every disease, and every ailment to a mineral deficiency." Dr. Henry Schroeder, M.D., Ph.D., of Dartmouth College, said, "Your mineral needs are even more important than your vitamin needs, since your body cannot make minerals." Good health is inextricably linked to vitamins *and* minerals. Consider this verbatim quote from the 74th Congress 2nd Session:

> *We know that vitamins are complex chemical substances which are indispensable to nutrition, and that each of them is of importance for normal function of some special structure in the body. Disorder and disease result from any vitamin deficiency. It is not commonly realized, however, that vitamins control the body's appropriation of minerals, and in the absence of minerals they have no function to perform. Lacking vitamins, the system can make some use of minerals, but lacking minerals, vitamins are useless.*

Ionic minerals are preferred. Make sure you take your vitamins *and* minerals regularly!

Nano Nano

One of the most exciting developments in the science of nutritional supplementation is the use of nanotechnology. A nano is one billionth of a metre and nanotechnology involves manufacture and manipulation of these extremely small structures. It was only in the 1980s that the instruments to view and manipulate these tiny bodies, which are much smaller than a molecule, were developed. Nanotechnologies offer huge advantages. Check this out . . .

Nanotechnology has given us the tools . . . to play with the ultimate toy box of nature—atoms and molecules . . . the possibilities to create new things appear to be limitless.

–Horst Stormer, Columbia University, Nobel Laureate

One of the world's leading centers in the Nanotechnology Revolution has been Rice University. In 1985, Rice professors Rick Smalley, Robert Curl, and Harold Kroto discovered the buckyball —a 60-carbon geodesic-shaped nanosize molecule that has been shown to be superconductive, promising advances in the control of electrons and many other benefits for mankind. In 1996, the Rice Team was awarded the Nobel Prize in Chemistry.

This breakthrough stimulated interest in nanotechnolgy at Rice, as an institution dedicated to the advancement of science. The university recognized the magnitude of this revolution and made a major commitment to it. Rice built a $30 million Center for Science and Nanoscale Technology, equipped with advanced instruments and staffed with 40 scientists from different fields. The school has encouraged outside industry to participate in development projects and holds seminars on nanotechnology.

*Four of the defining technologies of the 21st century will
be nanotechnology, biotechnology, information technology,
and environmental science. As a result, the potential both
for improving the quality and increasing the length of life
has never been greater.*

–Malcolm Gillis, President of Rice University

The U.S. alone is pouring about a billion dollars a year into nano research. At the time of this writing I am aware of only one company who is pioneering nanotechnology in nutritional supplements. Their products look very impressive indeed!

In Conclusion

From world-class athletes to weekend warriors to the rest of us, we all need to move our bodies regularly and often. Practice the 3 E's! Eat right, exercise right, and eliminate right—and that includes supplementing right! In addition, be sure to include the 3 R's: relax, rejuvenate, and rebalance. Premium-quality supplements make the difference in my life and they can in your life too!

Chapter Summary

The key ideas to remember are:

1. Every body needs to move regularly and often.

2. Use the three-step plan: assess now, make short-term goals, reassess results often.

3. ICAN: improvement, constant and never-ending (the law of increase).

4. Start small and simple and then *keep going*. Build on successes.

5. The 3 E's and the 3 R's are the foundation of excellent health.

6. Minerals are critical to health and ionic minerals are preferred.

7. Supplement with only the best products available such as sango coral calcium.

8. Check out nutritional supplements with nano-technology.

9. *I believe in you! You can do it!*

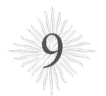

I Trust My Healthy Self

Health and improving one's health is a choice. We choose the level of health we experience every day, from moment to moment. If your health is optimum—if you wake each day totally energized and refreshed, if your emotions are fully charged, if you are as sharp as a razor mentally and creative, and you feel totally plugged into life and connected to the universe—then you are "normal." That's right, normal. That's what we are designed to feel. In today's world that would be considered outstanding and exceptional. Most people do not have that experience in a consistent way. In fact many people have much the opposite experience. That is common. Not normal, but common.

And what restores and optimizes our health? We must take the opposite path (or at least a different one!) than the one that brought us to the brink of this unprecedented un-wellness in the history of the world. Information and knowledge, motivation, action, and the reassessment of our priorities is a great place to begin. There is hope!

We must make changes and we must trust the innate wisdom of our bodies to heal and rejuvenate. It is natural to grow and change. It is necessary for the human spirit to want more. We must renew the trust within ourselves of our own abilities, and reclaim the responsibility for vibrant health. Trust yourself with a clear mind and an open heart. It can be done. It's not too late. The best time to begin is right now.

The Executive Summary

Here is the brief, no-frills, bare-to-the-bone, cut-to-the-chase executive summary for royal health!

1. 3 E's: eat right, exercise right, eliminate right.

2. 3 R's: relax, rejuvenate, rebalance.

3. AHA! Assess your present situation, be totally honest, and take consistent action.

4. Follow the acidity/alkalinity rules and eat 80/20.

5. Support your immune system with good digestion— stay alkaline!

6. Avoid acid-forming, non-nutritious foods including white flour products, pop, alcohol, processed foods, artificial foods and colours, preservatives, etc.

7. Choose healthful fats and oils and avoid refined ones.

8. Have a good sleep every night.

9. Cleanse (colon) at least annually and have regular daily eliminations.

10. Support your hormonal life naturally.

11. Stay fit and trim . . . do not become an overweight/ obese statistic.

12. Turn off your TV and get off the couch!

13. ICAN—improvement, constant and never-ending!

14. Look for nanotechnology products.

15. Everything counts!

16. Take premium-quality nutritional supplements that are made from organic sources.

17. Eat *organically produced* foods and eat lower on the food chain.

18. Shop locally as much as possible and eat in-season produce.

Get premium-quality nutritional supplements from exemplary companies. These are the commonly agreed upon essential nutrients:

+ *Macro minerals:* calcium, chloride, magnesium, phosphorous, potassium, sodium.

+ *Trace elements:* arsenic, boron, chromium, cobalt, copper, fluoride, iodine, iron, lead, lithium, manganese, molybdenum, nickel, selenium, silicon, vanadium, zinc.

+ *Vitamins:* A, B1, B2, B3, B5, B6, B12, C, D, E, K.

+ *Essential amino acids:* histidine, isoleucine, leucine, lysine, methionine, phenylalanine, threonine, tryptophan, valine.

+ *Essential fatty acids:* alpha-linolenic acid (n-3), linoleic acid (n-6).

For even more powerful supplementation consider adding spirulina, green food, wild yam (DHEA), phyto-nutrients, powerful antioxidants, aloe juice, CoQ10, DHA, sango coral calcium.

We hope you were reminded of things you already knew or that you learned something new. We hope we inspired you to take action for the sake of your health. Thank you for taking your time to read our book. It is our prayer that you live a long and healthy vibrant life!

Shine on!

Dawn and Robert

About the Authors

Dawn King

Dawn King is the queen of love and connection. With an uncanny knack for understanding people, coupled with a Ph.D. in street smarts and the gift of healing hands, Dawn has touched the lives of thousands of clients. For more than twenty years her unique approach to specialized kinesiology has seemed miraculous at times. In the domain of physical health she is especially gifted at relieving postural and chronic pain. Her amazing insights and understanding of human behaviour make her the consummate coach and mentor. Dawn has consistently provided outstanding and extraordinary results. As thousands of clients can testify, she is energetic, passionate, upbeat, slightly outrageous—and fun to be with! Dawn is a dedicated mother, wife, speaker, singer, tri-athlete, and author.

Robert King, M.Ed.

Robert King is a born teacher. With a master's degree in counselling and extensive training in behavioural therapies, Robert has enjoyed working with countless children, adults, and families. He comes from a lineage of respected writers and authors. With more than 25 years as a teacher/counselor, Robert shares a passion and a purpose of educating and inspiring people worldwide to live a healthy and vibrant life! His youthfulness and outstanding health are a result of his commitment to an exceptional healthy lifestyle. He is a man who walks his talk. Robert is a devoted father, hus-band, marathoner, musician, songwriter, and author.

Contact Information

Dawn and Robert King love to entertain, educate, and empower. Travel and meeting new people fuels their passion for living a vibrant life! Please contact them for available dates for:

- ✦ Keynote addresses
- ✦ Presentations
- ✦ Seminars
- ✦ Consultations

They always appreciate hearing from others, whether it is to order books or products, arrange appointments, presentations, or seminars, or just say hello. Although they have very busy schedules, they always do their best to respond promptly.

Dawn and Robert King may be contacted by:
Telephone: 250.545.7777 ✦ 1.877.295.5464 (toll-free)
Fax: 250.545.7732
Mail: P.O. Box 1720, Vernon, B.C. Canada, V1T 8C3

You may also visit their website:
www.DawnandRobertKing.com

Please contact Dawn or Robert King for more information regarding bulk order special pricing, other books and audio products, seminars, speaking, or consulting.

Order Form

Please send me _____ copy/copies of *Live a Vibrant Life* at $_____ per book. Enclosed is payment for:

Books	$ _____	
Shipping	$ _____	(*contact us first for shipping costs*)
Subtotal	$ _____	
Sales tax	$ _____	(6% Canadian residents only)
Total	$ _____	

Ship-to Address

Name _____

Organization _____

Address _____

_____

Phone _____

E-mail _____

Method of Payment

❏ Personal cheque or money order enclosed.

❏ Credit card   Type _____ Exp. _____

   Credit card # _____

Fax this form to: 250.545.7732
Or mail to: P.O. Box 1720, Vernon, B.C. Canada, V1T 8C3
Telephone: 250.545.7777 ✦ 1.877.295.5464 (toll-free)
website: www.DawnandRobertKing.com